Also from Jan Moran

Praise for *Scent of Triumph* (St. Martin's Griffin)

Now in Audiobook and ebook

"A haunting, multilayered historical romance, Jan Moran's *Scent of Triumph* is an epic journey. A book to savor, like the most beautiful of perfumes. Inhale. Exhale. I was riveted from start to finish...and I'm only just now finding my breath."
— Samantha Vérant, Author of *Seven Letters from Paris; A Memoir*

"A dedicated look into world of fashion; recommended."
— *Midwest Book Review*

"From war-torn Europe to the sunny climes of Southern California, *Scent of Triumph* is a captivating tale of love, loss, determination and reinvention. A page-turner."
— Karen Marin, Givenchy Paris

"Hard to put down...captivating. The tragedies of war, conflicts in family, love, and passion for perfumery paint a realistic, historical portrait of some of the fragrance industry's most famous women who created today's top cosmetic firms. A "must read" for anyone in cosmetics."
— Marvel Fields, Chairman Emeritus, American Society of Perfumers

"A gripping World War II story of poignant love and devastating, heart-wrenching loss. Perfumes are so beautifully described."
— Gill Paul, Author of *The Affair*

"A sweeping saga of one woman's journey through WWII. A heartbreaking, evocative read!"
— Anita Hughes, Author of *Lake Como*

"Action, suspense and romance as it follows its intrepid heroine through the turbulent years of World War II, from the depths of tragedy to the heights of success. Fragrance lovers will enjoy the skillful way in which scent is woven into the story…and how the heroine's experiences are filtered through her highly refined sense of smell."
– Nancy Arnott, A&E Television Networks

The Winemakers (St. Martin's Griffin)

"Beautifully layered and utterly compelling." — Jane Porter, *New York Times* & *USA Today* Bestselling Author

"Readers will devour this page-turner as the mystery and passions spin out." – *The Library Journal*

"Moran weaves knowledge of wine and winemaking into this intense family drama." – *Booklist*

"Spellbound by the thread of deception."
– The Mercury News

The *Love, California* Series
Empowering Romance with a Touch of Suspense

"A captivating world of glamour, romance, and intrigue."
— Melissa Foster, *New York Times* & *USA Today* Bestselling Author

"Jan Moran is the new queen of the epic romance."
— Rebecca Forster, *USA Today* Bestselling Author

"Jan rivals Danielle Steel at her romantic best."
— Allegra Jordan, author of *The End of Innocence*.

"Flawless is an astute, intelligent, gripping romance for the modern woman that offers a glimpse of glamour while showing those who work hard behind the scenes to create that glamour. The characters reach out and pull you into their lives and stay with you long after you close the book."
— Hannah Fielding, Author of *The Echoes of Love*

"Jan Moran's heroines are strong women who have made their way into the beauty world, and have the mental acuity to go head-to-head against the obstacles that fall in their path. They care deeply for their families and for their friends. They love with great sensuality. Fast-paced and well written, a major contender in the Women's Fiction market for just cause. Runway receives a strong five-star rating."
— Karen Laird, *Under the Shade Tree Reviews*

Vintage Perfumes

by

Jan Moran

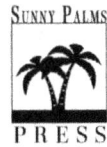

Copyright © 2015 by Jan Moran
All Rights Reserved.

All rights reserved under International and Pan-American Copyright Conventions, including the right of reproduction in whole or in part in any form or by any electronic or mechanical means including information storage and retrieval systems, without written permission, except in the case of brief quotations embodied in critical articles and reviews.

Library of Congress Cataloging-in-Publication Data
Moran, Jan.
/ by Jan Moran
Second edition

ISBN 978-1-942073-23-9 (softcover)
ISBN 978-1-942073-25-3 (epub ebooks)

Disclaimer: In this book we have relied on information provided by third parties and have performed reasonable verification of facts. We assume no responsibility or liability for the accuracy of information contained in this book. No representations or warranties, expressed or implied, as to the accuracy or completeness of this book or its contents are made. The information in this book is intended for entertainment purposes only, and the characters are entirely fictional. Every effort has been made to locate the copyright holders of materials used in this book. Should there be any errors or omissions, we shall be pleased to make acknowledgements in future editions.

Printed in the U.S.A.
Cover design by Silver Starlight Designs
Cover images copyright 123RF

For Inquiries Contact:
Sunny Palms Press
9663 Santa Monica Blvd., Suite 1158
Beverly Hills, CA, USA
www.SunnyPalmsPress.com
www.JanMoran.com

Other Books by Jan Moran

20th Century Historical

The Winemakers: A Novel of Wine and Secrets
Scent of Triumph: A Novel of Perfume and Passion
Life is a Cabernet: A Companion Wine Novella to The Winemakers

Contemporary

The Love, California Series:
Flawless
Beauty Mark
Runway
Essence
Style
Sparkle

NonFiction

Vintage Perfumes
Fabulous Fragrances
Fabulous Fragrances II

Browse her entire collection at www.JanMoran.com
Get a free ebook when you join Jan's VIP list.

Introduction

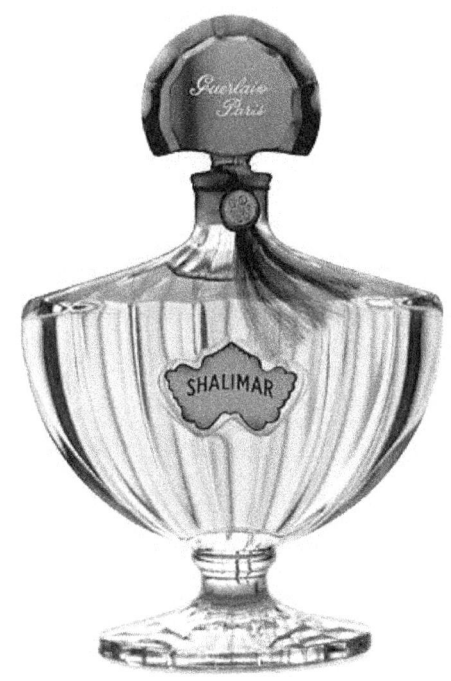

IN WRITING *Vintage Perfumes*, one of the most difficult aspects of planning this book was selecting the perfumes for inclusion. At first, I approached this task in a strict manner—*nothing after 1950*, I told myself. But how could I not include some of the magnificent masterpieces from the mid-1950s, such as Diorissimo?

Once again, I was quite firm with myself. Nothing after 1960. But how could I leave out Bal à Versailles or Chant d'Arômes? *Impossible.*

Of course, 1970 would really be stretching the boundary, but then...what about 1000 by Jean Patou? Or Cabochard and Cristalle? These perfumes are legends.

I finally drew the line at 1980, more or less. Too new, you might wonder? Consider this: A fragrance created in 1980 is thirty-five years old as of this writing. Granted, most of the perfumes in this book are pre-1950, but I felt the collection would be incomplete without including perfumes that have reached the legendary status. I hope you find your beloved perfumes in this collection, along with a few more to try and cherish.

The fragrances included in this book are generally available somewhere in the world. However, perfume brands often come and go, perhaps some by the time you read this, so a few might have been discontinued. On the other hand, I applaud companies that are reintroducing vintage perfumes. While regulations and scarcity of ingredients may prohibit strict adherence to original formulas, know that perfumers work hard to recreate vintage perfumes.

In my previous book, *Fabulous Fragrances*, feminine and masculine fragrances were divided, but this time you'll find them combined. Many fragrances—particularly vintage brands—are unisex, but I've also found that people have learned to wear what they like regardless of whether a fragrance is marketed to men or women. Many women wear

Dior's fascinating citrus scent, Eau Sauvage, while many men have discovered the wooded magnificence of Patou's 1000.

In the years that have passed since I first wrote *Fabulous Fragrances*, my work veered into the technology arena. *Fabulous Fragrances* became the genesis for an innovative idea, which eventually became a touch-screen fragrance finder called Scentsa. This innovation won a FiFi award from The Fragrance Foundation and found a home in Sephora stores in the U.S., Canada, France, Denmark, Mexico, and Brazil, as well as in DFS stores in Hong Kong and Abu Dhabi. Once the product was established, Sephora acquired the technology so I returned to my passion of writing. Scentsa is now known as FragranceIQ and SkinIQ at Sephora stores.

Shortly thereafter, St. Martin's Press published my historical novel, aptly named *Scent of Triumph: A Novel of Perfume and Passion*. The saga is about a female French perfumer during World War II, and in it you'll find many references to vintage perfumes and perfumers of the period. I loved researching this story and focusing on the olfactory sense. You'll find an excerpt in the back of this book.

Thank you for reading and sharing your love of vintage perfume with others, and I hope you continue to find joy in the world of vintage perfumery.

-Jan Moran

Contents

Introduction 9
Vintage Perfumery 21
Vintage Style 25
The Perfumes 29
1000 29
4711 31
Acqua di Parma Colonia 33
Adieu Sagesse 35
Aliage 36
Aloha Tiaré (Tiaré) 37
Amazone 38
Anaïs Anaïs 40
Après L'Ondée 42
Aramis 44
Aria di Capri 45
Aromatics Elixir 46
Arpège 48
Azurée 49
Bal à Versailles 51
Bandit 53
Bellodgia 55
Bijan Perfume for Women 56

JAN MORAN

Blue Grass 58

Bois de Cédrat 59

Bois des Îles 61

Cabochard 62

Calandre 64

Calèche 66

Capricci 67

Chaldée 68

Chamade 70

Chanel No. 5 72

Chanel No. 18 74

Chanel No. 19 75

Chanel No. 22 77

Chant d'Arômes 79

Chantilly 80

Cinnabar 81

Citrus Bigarrade 83

Climat 84

Cocktail 85

Coco 86

Cœur Joie (Coeur Joie) 88

Colony 89

Cristalle 90

Vintage Perfumes

Cuir de Russie 92

Diorama 93

Diorella 94

Dioressence 96

Diorissimo 97

Diorling 98

Eau d'Hadrien 99

Eau d'Hermès 101

Eau d'Orange Verte 102

Eau de Camille 103

Eau de Campagne 104

Eau de Cologne 105

Eau de Cologne du Coq 106

Eau de Cologne Impériale 107

Eau de Guerlain 109

Eau de Patou 110

Eau Sauvage 111

En Avion 112

Epicéa 114

Estée 114

Fantasia de Fleurs 116

Farouche 117

Femme 118

Fidji 120
Fille d'Eve 121
Fiori di Capri 122
First 123
Fleurissimo 125
Fleurs de Bulgarie 126
Fleurs de Rocaille 127
Folavril 128
Fracas 130
Gardénia 132
Gardénia Passion 133
Giorgio 134
Givenchy III 136
Green Irish Tweed 137
Habanita 138
Habit Rouge 139
Indiscret 140
Infini 143
Ivoire 144
Je Reviens 146
Jicky 147
Joy 149
Kiehl's Original Musk 152

Vintage Perfumes

L'Air du Temps 153
L'Heure Attendue 155
L'Heure Bleue 156
L'Interdit 158
Lauren 159
Lavanda Imperiale 160
Le Dix 161
Liù 163
Ma Griffe 164
Magie Noire 166
Mediterraneo Carthusia 167
Miss Dior 168
Mitsouko 170
Mouchoir de Monsieur 172
Mûre et Musc 173
My Sin 175
N'Aimez Que Moi 176
Nahéma 177
Narcisse Noir 179
Normandie 180
Nuit de Noël 182
Old Spice 183
Ombre Rose 185

Opium 186
Oscar 188
Paloma Picasso Mon Parfum 190
Paris 192
Parure 193
Passion 195
Pavlova 196
Polo 197
Pour Une Femme 199
Private Collection 200
Que sais-je? 201
Quelques Fleurs L'Original 202
Rive Gauche 203
Rose Absolue 205
Royal Secret 206
Shalimar 207
Sikkim 210
Soir de Paris (Evening in Paris) 211
Sous Le Vent 212
Spanish Leather 213
Tabac Blond 215
Vanille (Vanille Passion) 216
Vent Vert 218

Vintage Perfumes

Vetiver 219

Visa 220

Vol de Nuit 222

White Linen 223

White Shoulders 225

Wind Song 226

Y 227

Youth Dew 228

Zeste Mandarine Pamplemousse 229

Common Ingredients 231

Bibliography and Sources 247

Vintage Perfumes Book Club Discussion 253

Excerpt from *Scent of Triumph* Novel 255

Scent of Triumph Book Club Discussion 283

Scent of Triumph AromaTrack 285

Contact Us 287

About the Author 289

Vintage Perfumery

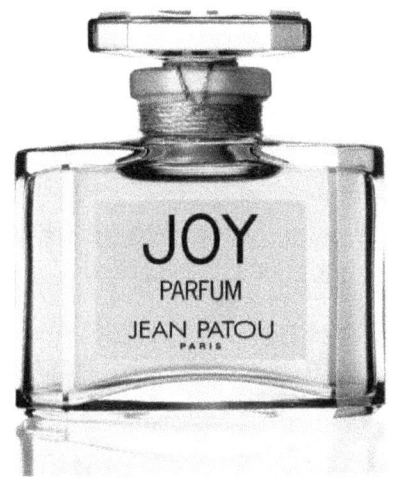

IN VINTAGE PERFUMERY, one of the most frequent complaints from users is a sense that the formula has changed, and indeed, that is often the case. There are several reasons for this.

First, to maintain a fragrance unchanged over time is a challenge for both art and science. For example, the scent of jasmine differs from field to field and from year to year depending on climate, rainfall, and soil conditions. The chemist must tweak the formula to compensate for changes in ingredients. In order to preserve the original perfume formulas, the French have established a library at the Osmathèque near Versailles.

Next, many ingredients have ceased to exist in the quantities needed for mass distribution. Perfumers are forced to recreate the fragrance from available ingredients.

Finally, governmental regulations have restricted the use of certain ingredients once used in original formulas. Reasons for restrictions include cruelty to animals and allergens. For example, civet from the civet cat and musk from the male musk deer are no longer allowed. In the European Union, potential allergens, such as oakmoss, have also been removed from formulas. In this book, these notes, or impressions, have been left in, because perfumers generally try to replicate these notes by using or blending other ingredients.

What else comprises vintage perfumes? Fine fragrances are created from essential oils present in plants, flowers, fruits, bark, roots, and other ingredients from the perfumer's palette. In Grasse, France, the center of the perfume industry, workers rise early to pick jasmine before dawn. When the sun peeks over the horizon, the flower loses twenty percent of its aroma. A skilled harvester can pick about a pound of flowers in forty-five minutes, or five thousand tiny blossoms. But only a few drops of essence will emerge after processing. Eight hundred pounds of jasmine flowers, or four million flowers, yield just one pound of concentrated oil. And the price for these essences? One pound of this oil, called jasmine absolute, will fetch from $10,000 to $20,000 or more, depending on

Vintage Perfumes

quality, while rose absolute can cost as much as $6,000 per pound.

Indian sandalwood must mature for thirty to fifty years before harvesting. Three thousand pounds of bergamot fruit from Calabria, Italy will yield only two pounds of essence. Now consider that many perfumes have hundreds of different essential oils, and it's clear that the precious artistry and gifts of nature that go into each bottle are staggering.

Natural essences are often blended with laboratory-created ingredients from natural or chemical compounds. A synthetic may be created as an imitation of a natural aroma, or as an entirely new aroma. Synthetics are far from being unworthy substitutes for nature; many are more tenacious and costly than natural ingredients. The aldehydes in Chanel No. 5 are an example. And whereas only a few hundred fragrances are available to perfumery from nature, synthetic fragrances offer the perfumer thousands. The combinations available today to the perfumer are virtually unlimited.

In fact, a perfumer might blend several components to give the impression of an ingredient, either to improve upon nature, or recreate an aroma that nature might not yield to perfumery. It is the essential oil, or combination of oils, that evokes an aroma, be it woody, spicy, floral, or something else.

A floral perfume may contain rose, violet, or sandalwood. Or it may not; perhaps it has been created by a combination of natural or synthetic materials that evokes such an aroma. This is how perfumers re-create the scent of the stubborn violet, which jealously refuses to yield its floral essence. The perfumer uses orris root from the iris, which has an aroma similar to that of violet and often exudes a powdery finish. Apricot is another example. Also re-created synthetically is musk—its source in nature is the male musk deer.

To keep a vintage brand alive is a challenge, from securing ingredients or replicating a beloved formula to keeping the brand relevant to contemporary buyers.

For more guidance on specific ingredients, turn to the back of this book for Commonly Used Ingredients in Perfumery. For the unusual component not listed consult a perfumery encyclopedia or search online for more information.

While there are many exquisite perfumes no longer being made, for the purpose of this book only perfumes that can still be purchased (besides vintage bottles) are included to limit the frustration of searching for perfumes no longer on the market.

Vintage Style

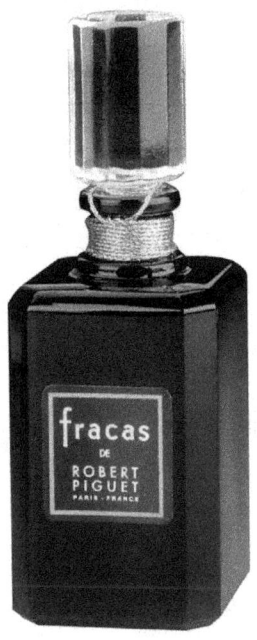

LIKE ANY WORK of art, literature, or fashion, perfume reflects the period in which it was created. From ancient times through today, fragrance has mirrored the mood of the period. Historical records show that the Greeks, Romans, Egyptians, Arabs, Persians, and Asians produced scents for bathing, religious rituals, banquets, entertaining, and medicinal purposes.

Modern perfumery began in the seventeenth-century in

the French town of Grasse where glovemakers used essences from the region's flowers and plants to scent gloves. At that time, leather was cured in a solution that gave it an unsavory smell. Perfume was used to mask this unpleasant odor, and scented gloves soon became the rage.

The eighteenth and nineteenth centuries witnessed expanded fragrance usage. Proper ladies wore lightly scented, single note fragrances. Lavender, violet, and rose were favored. Empress Josephine loved rose water, while Marie Antoinette went to her scaffold death with two vials of Houbigant perfume ensconced in her bosom for courage. Men and women wore similar fragrances. It was the marketing-savvy merchants of the twentieth-century who began to promote fragrances designed for each gender.

The early twentieth-century introduced rapid technological advances, winds of social change, and daring new fashions. Heretofore scandalous multi-floral scents became popular, as did spicy Oriental blends. In the 1920s and 1930s chemists experimented with new formulas, using synthetic ingredients to create classic scents that are still with us. The mood was expansive. Woolworth heiress Barbara Hutton, actresses Mary Pickford and Constance Bennett, and thousands of others snapped up Joy, which was introduced as the costliest perfume in the world. Couturiers branded perfume with their own labels: Coco Chanel, Paul Poiret, Jeanne Lanvin, Jean Patou, and Charles Worth. Some early designer perfumes have survived, but most have not.

Vintage Perfumes

During World War II, few perfumers continued to work, and little remains from this period except for Fracas and Bandit. The late 1940s and 1950s saw a return to feminine floral fragrances, complementing the flowing skirts and tiny waists of Christian Dior's New Look fashions. Estée Lauder sparked demand in the United States for everyday perfume when she launched Youth Dew in 1953. Gloria Swanson, Joan Crawford, Dolores Del Rio, and the Duchess of Windsor praised the striking Oriental fragrance. Youth Dew's blockbuster appeal did not go unnoticed by the large cosmetic and fragrance companies. The ensuing decades saw larger budgets, mega-launches, and more designer imprints than ever.

Social upheaval marked the 1960s and 1970s: the sexual revolution, civil rights, and women's rights movement. Fragrance reflected these changes with bold new scents rich with musk and patchouli. The greed-is-good eighties traded in glitz, intrigue, sex, and money with fragrance hits like Opium, distinctive, heady scents with rediscovered Oriental, or spicy, essences. The designer race was also ablaze. Couturier names were recognizable, marketable, and they also wanted a piece of the action.

Fifty years from now, new and contemporary brands will be considered vintage, and like their predecessors, these perfumes will also reflect the fashions and culture of the time.

The Perfumes

1000

Jean Patou

Jean Kerléo, the in-house master perfumer for Jean Patou, favors the precious essence of jasmine and rose he used in abundance in 1000, or Jean Patou Mille. The company describes the fragrance as "the essence of extravagance," a costly formula born of mostly natural ingredients.

The addition of violet, iris, and aromatic woods is designed to endow the wearer with an aura of wealth, breeding, and good taste. The perfume moves through a variety of stages, from the bright aldehydic and fresh green opening to the voluptuous iris, jasmine, and rose bouquet. The silky wooded finish of patchouli, incense, and sandalwood reveals a richly detailed inner life, reminiscent of scenes from Dora Levy Mossanen's book, *Harem*.

Wear it to close an important business deal or to a glamorous affair—or simply to feel indulgent. Elegant, glamorous, and refined, it is a fragrance that moves gracefully through a variety of seasons and occasions. Another timeless creation from the House of Patou.

Jan's Note: The earlier, pre-EU version of 1000 was drier in character while today's reformulated edition brings forth the rich bouquet of jasmine and rose just a little more—although the slightly mysterious wooded finish still melds beautifully with the skin.

A robustly glamorous perfume, 1000 is that timeless little black dress in your closet, the one you reach for when nothing less than elegance will do. But don't let that dissuade you from wearing 1000 with the perfect white shirt and jeans. Like a designer handbag, it will instantly elevate your style, giving you a certain *je ne sais quoi* sure to turn heads in your confident wake.

Scent Type: Floral
Top Notes: Greens, bergamot, anjelica, coriander, tarragon
Heart Notes: Chinese osmanthus, jasmine, rose, lily of the valley, violet, iris, geranium
Base Notes: Vetiver, patchouli, moss, sandalwood, amber, musk, civet

Who's Worn It
Jacqueline Kennedy Onassis, Bianca Jagger, Angelica Huston, Andrea Marcovicci, Teri Garr

Vintage Perfumes

Introduced: 1972

***

4711

Muelhens

The original 4711 Eau de Cologne formula was first produced in eighteenth-century Germany. Invigorating citrus top notes create a tart, stimulating scent, followed by light florals and warm, exotic woods. It is a refreshing, sporty fragrance worn by women and men. Indeed, many of the herbs used in 4711 have been used historically as external application for headaches and rejuvenation, though we can't vouch for their effectiveness.

The dominant note in 4711 is bergamot, which is a tangy fresh oil derived from an inedible citrus fruit. Perfumers tell us the best bergamot trees in the world are in Calabria, Italy. Bergamot is often found in the top notes of fragrances, especially eaux de cologne. An excellent fixative, it is also the prime ingredient in Earl Grey tea.

The history of 4711 is as rich as the fragrance. A Carthusian monk reputedly developed the eighteenth-century formulation before the formula came into the hands of German businessman Ferdinand Muelhens, who began marketing the cologne. When the French descended upon Germany in that century, they renumbered street addresses. The businessman found himself with a new address, Glockengasse No. 4711, Köln, a number he adopted for the cologne. The name and the scent have endured.

The elegantly tooled label remains unchanged. The cologne is housed in a handsome gold-colored bottle, embellished with turquoise lettering.

Jan's Note: In a word: simplicity. This classic eau de cologne has stood the test of time. *Why?* you might wonder, especially when there are so many other exquisite citrus splashes from the most exclusive brands in perfumery. But that's precisely the reason. The classic 4711 is a straightforward eau de cologne, an economical energizing splash made for your personal daily routine.

Like your morning coffee or tea, the bracing brightness of 4711's lemon, lavender, and rosemary blend will help recharge your morning battery. After this light scent vaporizes around noon, you can move on to more complex fragrances.

Scent Type: Chypre - Fresh
Top Notes: Bergamot, orange oil, lemon, basil, peach
Heart Notes: Bulgarian rose, jasmine, melon, lily, cyclamen, lavender, rosemary
Base Notes: Haitian vetiver, Indian sandalwood oakmoss, patchouli, cedarwood, musk

Vintage Perfumes

Who's Worn It
Queen Victoria of England, Johann Wolfgang von Goethe, Richard Wagner

Introduced: 1792

***

Acqua di Parma Colonia
Acqua di Parma

Much to the dismay of fragrance lovers the world over, Acqua di Parma Colonia, favorite of the silver screen set and other icons of style, languished for years in the marketplace in relative obscurity. Then, to the delight of many, new ownership breathed renewed life into this magnificent unisex scent. A dynamic trio of style setters—Diego Della Valle of J.P. Tod's, Paolo Borgomanero of La Perla, and Luca di Montezemolo of Ferrari—have revived this popular Italian classic.

Acqua di Parma Colonia, literally translated as "water of Parma," is a brisk citrus cologne with lavender overtones and a rosy heart. It is packaged in apothecary-style bottles ensconced in sunny yellow boxes. Crisp and cool and undeniably sexy with a streak of chic. Wear it anytime to keep your cool. Imagine yourself in the 1950s, in dark sunglasses and Capri pants, taking a leisurely stroll overlooking the magical Italian coast. That's Acqua di Parma Colonia.

Additions to the Acqua di Parma line include Lavanda

Tonica, a lavender formulation for women and men, and Profumo, the company's first fragrance made exclusively for women—an intense potion of eighty percent jasmine. Finally, for aromatherapy aficionados, try the company's Blu Mediterraneo line.

Jan's Note: Acqua di Parma Colonia is one of those sunny fragrances I reach for when I want to close my eyes for a moment and imagine myself relaxing on the Italian Riviera. Its brisk citrus beginning warms to a powdery sensation that lingers on the skin, unlike lighter weight eaux de cologne.

The bright verbena note is clean and warm—less abrasive than stark, slap-your-face lemon. Perhaps for this reason, I'm a fan of the soaps and body lotions in this line—or maybe it's because a well-scented bath is one of life's little luxuries.

Scent Type: Citrus
Notes: Citrus, verbena, lavender, rose

Who's Worn It
Audrey Hepburn, Isabella Rossellini, Ava Gardner, Sandra Bullock, Cary Grant, David Niven, Kate Moss, Sharon Stone

Introduced: 1916
***

Vintage Perfumes

Adieu Sagesse
Jean Patou

Adieu Sagesse is the third fragrance of French couturier Jean Patou's love trilogy, along with Amour Amour and Que sais-je? Adieu Sagesse was created to commemorate the third stage of love, the moment when the body surrenders to desire. In French, *adieu sagesse* means "farewell wisdom."

Patou envisioned this slightly spicy, tart floral for fiery redheads, though anyone can enjoy the mélange of light fruity top notes artfully blended with sensual base notes.

Legendary perfumer Henri Alméras created this vintage gem in 1925, and in 2014, the Jean Patou company brought back Adieu Sagesse as part of its Heritage Collection.

Jan's Note: I'm often asked about the perfumes in this Jean Patou trio; it seems people are intrigued about choosing a fragrance based on hair color. If you live your life according to your daily horoscope, go ahead—but really, anyone who likes a vintage feel can wear Adieu Sagesse.

Scent Type: Chypre Floral - Fruity
Top Notes: Neroli, jonquil, lily of the valley
Heart Notes: Carnation, tuberose, opopanax
Base Notes: Musk, civet

Who's Worn It

JAN MORAN

Tennis star Suzanne Lenglen

Introduced: 1925

***

Aliage

Estée Lauder

Aliage is one of the original sport fragrances for women. "[It] was an idea ahead of its time," states the Estée Lauder firm. Aliage is a green chypre blend of more than 300 ingredients from Estée Lauder. Reportedly the aroma of fresh palm leaves served as inspiration for the sporty scent, which Lauder created for casual active wear. It is said she was searching for a light fragrance suitable for a midday tennis game.

The remarkable story of Estée Lauder began with a skin treatment formula that spawned the signature line of color cosmetics, skin care and fragrance, as well as the Prescriptives, Clinique, Aramis, and Lauder for Men lines, along with a host of acquisitions. Other Lauder activities include the Estée and Joseph H. Lauder Foundation and the endowment of the Lauder Institute for International Studies at the Wharton School of Business, University of Pennsylvania. The Lauder empire serves as an enduring example of what one woman can accomplish when she follows her dreams and commits herself to an ideal.

Vintage Perfumes

Jan's Note: While I might not wear this for a steamy game of tennis as Lauder imagined, it's one I *would* wear after tennis or a day at the spa. Aliage is a fresh, foresty, great-outdoors sort of green fragrance. Subtle rose and peach plant this well-tuned fragrance firmly in the terra of classic chypre scents while galbanum and vetiver give Aliage its green cut-grass character. For those who can't wear flowery perfumes, this is an excellent, tasteful choice.

Scent Type: Chypre – Green
Top Notes: Greens, peach, citrus oils
Heart Notes: Jasmine, rosewood, pine, thyme
Base Notes: Oakmoss, musk, vetiver, myrrh, galbanum

Introduced: 1972

***

Aloha Tiaré (Tiaré)
Comptoir Sud Pacifique

Say aloha! Aloha Tiaré from the French firm of Comptoir Sud Pacifique is a Hawaiian tropical garden breeze that's fragrant, sweet, and sunny.

This 1976 classic portrays the Hawaiian isles with green frangipani leaves and a tiaré flower and ylang-ylang bouquet. Coconut, vanilla, and musk merge with delightful tropical flair. The result is a soft gardenia-style aroma.

Create a relaxing holiday frame of mind for island

daydreaming. Perfect for Maui moods; pair it with sandals and sarongs. Packaged in travel-ready aluminum bottles that won't break like glass in the suitcase.

Jan's Note: Wearing perfume should be fun, and that's exactly what you get with Aloha Tiaré. It's a casual, sweet island scent that I like to wear with a bare sundress on balmy evenings. It's a piña colada at sunset. Don't over think this one, just enjoy.

Scent Type: Classic Floral
Top Notes: Coconut
Heart Notes: Ylang-ylang, frangipani, tiare, monoï
Base Notes: Tahitian vanilla

Introduced: 1976

***

Amazone
Hermès

Amazone is from Hermès, the Parisian maker of fine leathers, silks, porcelains, fashions, and more since 1837. Amazone is a modern floral bouquet with lively top notes of fruity citrus, most notably orange, lemon, raspberry, and black currant bud. The delicate floral heart is formed with hyacinth, jasmine, and narcissus amid a proliferation of other floral essences. It is ideal for liberal daytime use.

Vintage Perfumes

Master perfumer Jean-Claude Ellena, who is the in-house perfumer for Hermès, calls it "a spirited and cheerful fragrance." In French, the vintage name refers to a horsewoman riding sidesaddle. Hermès also describes Amazone as "tender and impetuous," a playful fragrance full of romance and charm. A chic vintage find, Amazone was the second women's fragrance developed by Hermès.

Jan's Note: Amazone is a blue-blooded thoroughbred for those who want a polished, well-balanced perfume. If it seems to you that Amazone has changed over the years—you're correct. It's gone through a few iterations, but the current version is still quite well done. Perhaps a bit more green here, a lighter wooded finish there, but its essential character remains under the continued orchestration of a fine line of perfumers. It's rather like a lovely woman who subtly changes her look from year to year. All in all, Amazone is still beautifully refined.

Scent Type: Floral – Fruity/Woody
Top Notes: Lemon, orange, bergamot, peach, strawberry, grapefruit, tangerine, galbanum, black currant bud
Heart Notes: Daffodil, hyacinth, narcissus, black currant bud, iris, jasmine, rose, raspberry, lily of the valley
Base Notes: Sandalwood, nutmeg, vetiver, cedarwood, neroli, ylang-ylang, oakmoss

JAN MORAN

Who's Worn It
Tina Turner

Introduced: 1974

***

Anaïs Anaïs
Jean Bousquet

Anaïs Anaïs is a nostalgic floral blend, delicate, soft, and subtle. French couturier Jean Bousquet, founder of Cacharel, describes his fragrance in these words: "Anaïs Anaïs is a perfume whose essence is romanticism with the scent of lilies. It has been housed in opaque jars reminiscent of the ancient world." The white jars bear a peach floral motif, created by bottle designer Annegret Beier. Anaïs Anaïs is an ideal scent for the young and the young at heart, those who are gentle and feminine in nature.

The innocence of the scent is created by the dominant note of white lilies, called Madonna lilies, cultivated in the south of France, Bulgaria, and the Middle East. Greeks and Romans considered this lily a symbol of purity. Each lily produces a few drops of the precious essence; in fact, one ton of petals produces only one pound of lily oil.

Bousquet clearly takes pleasure in selecting interesting names. He borrowed the name of his company, Cacharel, from the wild ducks native to Provence. And Anaïs Anaïs? The fragrance is named after the Persian Goddess of Love.

Vintage Perfumes

Jan's Note: We all have favorite perfumes that remind us of a certain time in our lives. For many women, Anaïs Anaïs is that perfume. It's the fragrance of youth, of virginal purity. It's springtime in the Alps, with the *Sound of Music* soaring in the background, wildflowers swaying in the breeze. Remarkably unchanged over time, and still one of my favorites.

Scent Type: Floral – Fresh
Top Notes: White Madonna lily, black currant bud, hyacinth, lily of the valley, citrus
Heart Notes: Moroccan jasmine, Grasse rose, Florentine iris, Madagascar ylang-ylang, orange blossom, Bourbon vetiver, California cedarwood, Singapore patchouli, Yugoslavian oakmoss
Base Notes: Russian leather, musk

Who's Worn It
Jennifer Aniston, Kate Moss, Sophie Dahl, Lisa Kudrow, Claudia Schiffer

Introduced: 1978

***

Après L'Ondée
Guerlain

A graceful creation by renowned perfumer Jacques Guerlain, the company describes Après L'Ondée as "an inspired portrait of the most delicate imaginary flower." Elusively charming, fresh and sparkling, it is a refined floral bouquet with a sweet amber base and one of the finest examples of surviving vintage perfumes.

Après L'Ondée is one of more than 300 perfumes developed by the renowned House of Guerlain. For many years before the company was sold to Louis Vuitton Moet Hennessey (LVMH), Guerlain was the world's oldest family-operated fragrance and cosmetic company. Spanning five generations, it was founded in 1828 by doctor and chemist Pierre-François-Pascal Guerlain. The shop was first located on the rue de Rivoli in Paris, then moved to No. 15 rue de la Paix where young Guerlain created his hallmark—personalized fragrances in sync with the wearer's personality, fragrances that often lived for only one evening or event.

Writer Honoré de Balzac commissioned a custom-blended scent during the writing of *César Birotteau*, and Empress Eugénie named Guerlain perfumer to the Napoléonic court for which many Empire fragrances were created. In fact, Guerlain was appointed perfumer to most of the royal courts of Europe, including those of the Empress of Austria and the Queens of England, Spain, and Romania.

Vintage Perfumes

But back to Après L'Ondée... A rich powdery almond note sets the tone with the addition of iris, while vetiver and violet add a green dimension that lifts the perfume to the level of greatness. Après L'Ondée is an exquisite perfume that must be tried at least once. It's easy to fall in love with this enchanting floral arrangement.

Jan's Note: There's a reason Guerlain perfumes have stood the test of time, and one of those is Après L'Ondée. If you've worn Shalimar or L'Heure Bleue and have yet to try Après L'Ondée, your education is incomplete. This was one of the first (if not *the* first) formulations to use heliotropin, which is responsible for the sense of powdery almond. This is an expansive, sun-warmed saga meant to be savored for its eternal romance.

Scent Type: Floral – Ambery
Top Notes: Violet, bergamot, cassie, neroli
Heart Notes: Heliotropin, carnation, ylang-ylang, iris, rose, jasmine, mimosa, vetiver, sandalwood
Base Notes: Vanilla, musk, amber, heliotrope

Introduced: 1906

***

Aramis
Estée Lauder

Introduced in 1965, Aramis from Estée Lauder remains a favorite among men's fragrances. Created by Bernard Chant (who also created Cabochard), Aramis is a classic chypre, or mossy-woody composition, which is a category characterized by the marriage of citrus and oakmoss with the addition of spicy patchouli. Green leaves, thyme, and sage form a fresh herbal accord, and spices of clove and cardamom create a warm heart. A superb lingering base is blended from vetiver and sandalwood, and a distinct leathery impression adds fullness.

A perennial favorite made for men (but women wear it, too), Aramis is a classic leather chypre that has stood the test of time.

Jan's Note: Aramis is the dance partner of the original Cabochard (may it rest in peace). Don't be afraid to steal this one from your man's dresser on a crisp autumn morning—it has a rich feeling of warm suede and flannel. If you want, lighten it with a mist of something citrusy.

Though changed some over the years, Aramis is ripe for rediscovery.

Vintage Perfumes

Scent Type: Chypre
Top Notes: Citrus, green leaves, sage, thyme
Heart Notes: Clove, cardamom
Base Notes: Oakmoss, patchouli, vetiver, sandalwood

Who's Worn It
Ines de la Fressange, Susan Gutfreund, Karl Lagerfeld

Introduced: 1965

***

Aria di Capri
Carthusia

Fresh trade winds sweeten a wildflower bouquet in Aria di Capri, a legendary fragrance from the sunny island of Capri. The firm of Carthusia, working with noted perfumer Laura Tonatto, hand produces perfumes using ancient methods developed by Capri's order of Carthusian monks.

Aria di Capri is a refreshing blend for women that begins with bright lemon and orange. Mimosa and peach convey natural freshness, while bay leaves spice this song of scent.

According to legend, monks of the Carthusian Monastery of St. Giacomo blended the original Capri perfumes in the 14th century. In 1948, the Father Prior discovered the ancient formula. With the Pope's permission, production began. Today, the tiny perfumery of Carthusia produces its line in accordance with tradition using the island's natural flora and vintage methods.

"A fresh and vibrant scent, like Capri's sea breeze, warm sun and blue skies." - Carthusia

Jan's Note: Whether this fragrance is actually a vintage number—or merely channeling vintage style—is often debated, but as a writer, I believe in suspending disbelief and going with a good story. This one ends happily, too, with an airy floral infused with peach. Aptly named and worth a try.

Scent Type: Fresh Floral
Top Notes: Peach, Bay
Heart Notes: Mimosa, jasmine
Base Notes: Iris (orris)

Who's Worn It
Susan Sarandon

Introduced: 1948

***

Aromatics Elixir
Clinique

Aromatics Elixir is designed to soothe and subtly stimulate with notes of gentle chamomile and sweet sandalwood set against a classic blend of French florals and aromatic woods. The dominant chypre theme is a natural

Vintage Perfumes

accord enhanced by juicy citrus and lawn greens.

"For the individualist in every woman. Aromatics Elixir is an intriguing, rebellious fragrance. It touches the senses and spirit in subtle, pleasing ways with notes of rose, jasmine, ylang-ylang, and vetiver." – Clinique

Jan's Note: If you haven't tried master perfumer Bernard Chant's Aromatics Elixir, it's like nothing you would expect from a company with such a squeaky clean image. Although it sports a natural herbal mask, lurking beneath is a riot of sexy patchouli. Extraordinarily well done and entirely unique—if it's meant for you, you'll know it immediately.

Scent Type: Chypre - Floral
Top Notes: Chamomile, orange blossom, bergamot, coriander, rosewood, aldehydes, greens, palmarosa
Heart Notes: Jasmine, rose, ylang-ylang, tuberose, orris, carnation
Base Notes: Sandalwood, oakmoss, vetiver, patchouli, musk, cistus, civet

Who's Worn It
Glenn Close, Kate Blanchett

Introduced: 1971

***

Arpège
Lanvin

Arpège is a restoration and reformulation of the original 1927 scent from French couturier Jeanne Lanvin and perfumer Andre Fraysse.

More than sixty natural essences are housed in the classic Art Deco, ball-shaped flacon, or *boule noire*. A black opaque glass bottle houses the perfume, while the eau de parfum resides in a clear glass bottle. A gold-colored image by artist Paul Iribe of Jeanne Lanvin and her daughter, musician Marie-Blanche, dressing for a ball is stamped on the glass just as it was on the original bottles.

The fragrance was christened Arpège by Marie-Blanche for its similarity to a musical arpeggio—a tumble of notes in quick succession. The result is an elegant floral composition with a sensual wooded finish.

Lanvin created the popular mother-daughter design concept in addition to designing evening gowns, bridal wear, and menswear. After her death in 1946, Marie-Blanche, also known as the Comtesse de Polignac, continued the business with Bernard Lanvin.

The relaunch of Arpège coincided with the remodeling of Lanvin's boutiques on the rue du Faubourg Saint Honoré. Arpège is a classic revived.

Vintage Perfumes

Jan's Note: The once powdery, intensely romantic Arpège has now evolved into a more modern edition with a distinctly woody finish. Still refined, but different from what you might recall, like entering the redecorated Paris flat of a favorite aunt.

Scent Type: Woody Floral
Top Notes: Bergamot, aldehydes, peach, orange blossom, honeysuckle, iris
Heart Notes: Rose, jasmine, ylang-ylang, coriander, mimosa, tuberose, violet, geranium, genet
Base Notes: Sandalwood, vetiver, patchouli, vanilla, musk

Who's Worn It
Audrey Hepburn, Diana, Princess of Wales, Martha Stewart, Princess Grace of Monaco, Rita Hayworth, Jacqueline Bisset

Introduced: 1927

***

Azurée
Estée Lauder

Azurée is a chypre floral melody from Estée Lauder, said to have been inspired by the tangy Mediterranean bergamot fruit, an inedible fruit prized for perfumery.

Created by Bernard Chant, the perfumer who was

known for magnificent leathery floral compositions, Azurée remains faithful to the original vision of its creator.

The fragrance features herbal and aldehydic top notes, dry floral heart notes, and woody base notes redolent of warm leather and moss. Azurée is, quite simply, a grand perfume.

Jan's Note: As noted in the Aramis profile, Azurée was created by a talented perfumer who was known for robust leathery blends. Azurée has a dry, almost masculine character, along with a dusky feminine edge that's as muted as twilight, and wrapped in a sunny citrus halo. Though it has been relieved of its oakmoss, it's still an audacious, fearless crusader for the bold point of view.

Don't discount this well-priced, thinly promoted fragrance—Azurée has certainly earned its place among hall of fame classics.

Scent Type: Chypre
Top Notes: Bergamot, aldehydes, gardenia, artemisia
Heart Notes: Jasmine, geranium, ylang-ylang, orris, cyclamen
Base Notes: Leather, oakmoss, patchouli, musk, amber

Introduced: 1969

***

Vintage Perfumes

Bal à Versailles

Jean Desprez

Bal à Versailles is a classic French fragrance from the legendary Parisian perfumer Jean Desprez. More than 350 rare essences were used to create the long-lasting, dramatic fragrance. A rich and feminine Oriental blend, it features floral, amber, spice, and sweet balsamic base notes. Bal à Versailles is ideal for sophisticated day wear and elegant evenings.

In the 1930s, Jean Desprez established his perfumery on the prestigious rue de la Paix in Paris serving an exclusive clientele. Besides his popular Bal à Versailles, he also created Grand Dame, Étourdissant, and Vôtre Main in 1939, Jardanel in 1972, and Révolution à Versailles. Upon his death in 1973, he was succeeded by his son Denis Desprez and daughter Marie Celine Garnier.

Bal à Versailles is presented in an array of classic fragrance flacons. Our favorite is a round decanter with a label featuring a romantic party scene; no doubt it is from the most famous dance or "ball" of Versailles, the Bal à Versailles. This scene is a miniature reproduction of a Fragonard painting that is part of the Sevres Museum collection. The scene also appeared on a porcelain dish by Madame Ducluzeau known as *La Coupe des Sens*, or "cup of the senses," featuring miniatures representing the five senses. When Desprez was searching for inspiration, he spied the cup and was intrigued by the Fragonard scene representing the sense of smell. *Quel appropos!*

Jan's Note: Although Bal à Versailles has undergone a few facelifts, this powerhouse of glamour remains as daring as ever. Though the packaging has changed, the seductive force within remains close to the original, yet with edited base notes.

When I was researching the legendary Bal à Versailles, I came across reports that both Elizabeth Taylor and Michael Jackson loved Bal à Versailles. Knowing that they were close friends, it didn't surprise me that they shared a perfume as well. Dame Elizabeth instinctively knew how to project glamour—you might say Bal à Versailles was in perfect alignment.

Scent Type: Oriental - Ambery Spicy
Top Notes: Grasse jasmine, Bulgarian rose, Anatolian rose, May rose, Farnesian cassie
Heart Notes: Sandalwood, patchouli, vetiver
Base Notes: Musk, ambergris, gums, resins, civet

Who's Worn It
Dame Elizabeth Taylor, Michael Jackson

Introduced: 1962
***

Vintage Perfumes

Bandit

Robert Piguet

Bandit is a classic fragrance developed during World War II for couturier Robert Piguet by Roure perfumer Germaine Cellier. It is a delightfully wicked blend of sultry spices and florals with a long-lasting base of woods and musk, and the interesting addition of a bitter leathery note that adds a dark, mysterious, film noir impression. This is the original 1944 formula, resurrected in 1999, heretofore unavailable for twenty-five years.

Swiss-born Piguet apprenticed under couturier Paul Poiret in glamorous 1920 Paris. By 1928 he had his own salon specializing in couture creations for petite, youthful women. He trained the next generation of designers at his salon: Pierre Balmain, Hubert de Givenchy, Castillo, James Galanos. Christian Dior once said that he learned from Piguet "the virtues of simplicity...how to suppress." Piguet is often credited with "the little black dress."

Piguet was a man with a rebel heart, both in design and by action. In 1944, he introduced Bandit in a provocative manner with runway models in black bandit masks brandishing toy guns and knives. Remember, this was 1944. During the German occupation of France, Piguet defied Nazi orders to relocate to Berlin, remaining in Paris, in business, for the duration of World War II.

Born in 1909, Germaine Cellier was one of the first

female perfumers of the period. Known for daring, bold perfume compositions, Cellier was a master of distinctive artistry. Also known for blending Fracas, another Piguet fragrance, Cellier was an outspoken force who pushed the boundaries of conventional perfumery. Though she passed away in 1976, her masterpieces live on today, loved by legions.

Jan's Note: Though edited from the original formula due to the lack of vintage ingredients, Bandit remains black-and-white film noir, a throaty Marlene Dietrich clad in midnight black, a seductive smile barely touching her lips. A magnificently dry, leathery blend, Bandit is the exact opposite of its sister perfume, Fracas, which is a bold explosion of tuberose. Bandit is crimson autumn leaves, roaring fires, and dry Bordeaux.

Scent Type: Chypre – Leathery Floral
Top Notes: Neroli, orange, ylang-ylang, galbanum
Heart Notes: Jasmine, rose, tuberose, leather
Base Notes: Patchouli, mousse de chêne, vetiver, musk

Who's Worn It
Marlene Dietrich

Introduced: 1944
***

Vintage Perfumes

Bellodgia

Caron

Bellodgia is a classic 1920s fragrance from the notable French fragrance house Parfums Caron. The fragrance takes its name from a romantic island on Lake Como in Northern Italy. The feminine floral bouquet is distinguished by a rich accord of rose and jasmine accenting the dominant theme of spicy carnation. Bellodgia is a chic, sophisticated perfume.

Parfums Caron was established in Paris in 1904 to introduce fragrances created by master perfumer Ernest Daltroff. Today, Parfums Caron presents its timeless fragrances on the fashionable avenue Montaigne in Paris. The store is a sight to behold; each exquisite Caron fragrance is suspended in Louis XV-style Baccarat crystal flacons, from which customers can draw a desired amount of fragrance. Elsewhere, look for Bellodgia prepackaged in perfume and eau de toilette fragrance strengths.

One final note on Bellodgia: The original spiciness was a product of clove, but due to restrictions on certain perfume ingredients, the clove note of isoeugenol has been replaced in reformulation. The result is a fresher lift in the opening accord with a hint of citrus. Though a little different, Bellodgia is still evocative of a vintage era.

Jan's Note: Bellodgia conveys a feeling of vintage romance, rather like a faded love letter misted with time.

Scent Type: Floral
Top Notes: Lily of the valley
Heart Notes: Rose, jasmine, lily of the valley
Base Notes: Spicy carnation

Introduced: 1927

***

Bijan Perfume for Women
Bijan

A floral Oriental scent with soft top notes, Bijan Perfume for Women is the original signature fragrance from Bijan, prominent Beverly Hills menswear couture designer. "The woman who wears my fragrance is certainly not afraid to be noticed," says Bijan. "She is definitive about her personal style and is as sophisticated as she is alluring."

Two-and-a-half years in the making, the fragrance is composed of rich seductive florals poised against exotic woods, creating a refined, feminine statement that whispers of wealth. From kings to presidents to the simply well-to-do, Bijan's clients seek out his inimitable style at his "by appointment only" boutique in Beverly Hills.

The scent is packaged in a round bottle with a hole in the center. Designed by Bijan, the bottle garnered a 1993 Clear Choice Award from the Glass Packaging Institute. So exquisite is the bottle, Bijan created a custom-made chandelier for his Beverly Hills showroom using more than

Vintage Perfumes

one million dollars' worth of Bijan Perfume for Women bottles. "At night, when the light is on, the perfume in the bottles gives off the most gorgeous amber colors," explains Bijan. "It is magnificent!"

Jan's Note: A rich, cognac-colored perfume that reveals Bijan's Persian heritage with an ambery sheen as smooth as a silken tapestry. Glamour with a capital G.

Scent Type: Floral – Oriental
Top Notes: Ylang-ylang, narcissus, orange blossom
Heart Notes: Persian jasmine, Bulgarian rose, lily of the valley
Base Notes: Moroccan oakmoss, sandalwood, patchouli

Who's Worn It
Oprah Winfrey, Liza Minnelli, Natalie Cole, Hillary Clinton, Queen Elizabeth II, Anjelica Huston, Barbra Streisand, Annette Bening, Bo Derek, Candice Bergen, Whoopi Goldberg, Aretha Franklin, Teri Garr, Lesley Anne Warren

Introduced: 1986
***

Blue Grass
Elizabeth Arden

Blue Grass from Elizabeth Arden is an enduring, easy-to-wear classic ideal for casual, professional or daytime wear.

Elizabeth Arden was an early entrepreneur in the American cosmetics industry. Born Florence Nightingale Graham in Ontario, Canada, she derived her professional name from a favorite book: *Elizabeth and Her German Garden*. As a nurse, she developed a skin care regime that became popular in her beauty salons, the first of which opened its red door in New York in 1910.

Arden's love of nature and flowers inspired the name for Blue Grass after the shimmering view of verdant fields visible from the windows of her Virginia home where she also indulged her love of horses.

Rose, jasmine, and orange blossom bloom in the bountiful bouquet. A subtle hint of clove accents the rich Virginia cedarwood finish. Ultra-feminine and versatile, Blue Grass is perfectly paired with pearls and pumps or cotton khakis and sandals.

Treasure the timeless appeal of Blue Grass, a well-priced classic.

Vintage Perfumes

Scent Type: Powdery Floral
Top Notes: Aldehydes, lavender, orange, neroli, bergamot
Heart Notes: Jasmine, tuberose, narcissus, rose, carnation
Base Notes: Sandalwood, musk, tonka bean, benzoin

Who's Worn It
Queen Elizabeth II

Introduced: 1934

***

Bois de Cédrat
Creed

Fresh and zesty, Bois de Cédrat is a harmony of bright citrus fruits balanced with a subtle wooded finish. In this classic eau de cologne, brisk lemon and mandarin warm to a cedarwood finish on the skin. Invigorating and refined.

Created in 1875, Bois de Cédrat is an enduring vintage fragrance that can be worn by women or men with equal aplomb.

Jan's Note: The House of Creed dates from 1760, when founder James Henry Creed established his firm in London. Soon Creed fragrances were accepted into the inner circles of society including the French, Spanish, English, and Austro-Hungarian courts.

In 1854, the House of Creed moved to Paris and

continued to flourish under the tutelage of Creed descendants. More than two hundred fragrances later, sixth-generation perfumer Olivier Creed and his son carry on the family business. Creed custom designs scents for the firm's private clientele and also offers specialty fragrances to the public. All fragrances are handmade using a traditional infusion technique.

Creed's custom commissions remain exclusive to the client for five years, then the fragrance may be sold to the public. So who has indulged their fragrant passions? Fleurissimo was created for Princess Grace of Monaco's wedding day, Spring Flower was blended for Audrey Hepburn, and Impérial Millésime went to the King of Saudi Arabia. Royal English Leather was made for King George III, Orange Spice was created for Oscar Wilde, Tabarôme was made for Winston Churchill, and Royal Water was being developed for Diana, Princess of Wales, before she died.

Scent Type: Citrus
Notes: Lemon, mandarin, cedarwood

Who's Worn It
Georges Braque

Introduced: 1875
***

Vintage Perfumes

Bois des Îles
Chanel

In the 1920s, French couturier Gabrielle "Coco" Chanel collaborated with the great perfumer and Russian émigré to France, Ernest Beaux, to create the Chanel scents that have become legend: No. 5, No. 19, and No. 22. In 1993, Chanel reintroduced a trio of exhilarating Beaux fragrances from the twenties: Bois des Îles, Cuir de Russie, and Gardénia.

The woody floral blend of Bois des Îles begins with top notes of fresh citrus, spice, and sparkling aldehydes entwined with rich florals and woods, the star of which is sandalwood. A subtly sensual fragrance, an understated classic.

The main impression is one of sandalwood which is velvety soft, warm, and enticing. Spicy tonka bean vanillic balsams in the finish create a gingerbread-like impression, calling to mind the comfort of home on a wintry evening and the seduction of childhood sweets with a warm creamy glass of milk. Bois des Îles is a tactile fragrance of sweet reassurance, a warm cloak of class on a cool evening.

In creating Bois des Îles, Beaux was reportedly inspired by fellow Russian artists and their works, specifically composer Pyotr Ilyich Tchaikovsky and his opera *The Queen of Spades* (*La Dame de Pique*), which was based on a short story by novelist Aleksandr Pushkin. The lush fullness, deep notes, and hypnotic refrains are indeed an olfactory reminiscence of this 1890 opera.

Bois des Îles, or "wood of the isles," is a return to an era of grace and elegance. It is a stunning vintage masterpiece that remains forever ageless like the perfect little black Chanel dress.

Jan's Note: When I was in my early twenties I visited India and fell in love with the smooth, silky scent of sandalwood. As mercurial as moonlight, sandalwood is a multifaceted essence that adds warmth and depth to perfumes. In Bois des Îles, perfumer Ernest Beaux worked magic with sandalwood, and the result, even a century later, is still mesmerizing. If you like warm, complex aromas—such as the bouquet of a rich Bordeaux or a golden cognac—then Bois des Îles is not to be missed.

Scent Type: Spicy-Woody Oriental
Top Notes: Bergamot, petitgrain, coriander, aldehydes
Heart Notes: Jasmine, rose, ylang-ylang, iris
Base Notes: Vetiver, amber, sandalwood, tonka bean

Introduced: 1926

***

Cabochard
Grès

Originally introduced in 1959, and resurrected in 1972, the classic Cabochard from the Parisian House of Grès is a

Vintage Perfumes

soft, leathery chypre blend of citrus, mosses, and dry florals. Grès was born Alix Barton and became known for her fluid designs that draped the body. Twice she had to close her salon doors during World War II, but in 1946 she reestablished the House of Grès along with the fashions and the fragrances that remain with us today.

Legend has it that Grès had taken a trip through the Spice Islands and wished to re-create the olfactory experience. In response her perfumer, Bernard Chant, produced a scent evocative of fresh island greenery, citrus, herbs, tobacco, and leather. The result was Cabochard, the essence of the Spice Islands. The lingering essence is one of smoky leather, yet smoothly refined and highly original.

Although the reorchestration of Cabochard rendered the impression less dark and leathery and more earthy green, the result still harkens to a bygone era.

Jan's Note: Some people decry the new rendering of Cabochard, which is decidedly less dark and leathery while others find it refreshing. I always tell people to wear what they like, and you may well enjoy this version (although the original was utterly sublime). If you're expecting a smoky, ambery, leathery perfume, simply know that Cabochard has changed, and florals and fruits have been brought more to the foreground.

Scent Type: Chypre – Leather
Top Notes: Citrus, aldehydes, fruits, spices
Heart Notes: Jasmine, rose, ylang-ylang, orris, geranium
Base Notes: Leather, tobacco, amber, patchouli, musk, moss, vetiver, castoreum

Who's Worn It
Chynna Phillips

Introduced: 1959

***

Calandre
Paco Rabanne

Calandre is a classic fragrance from Spanish designer Paco Rabanne who dressed stars such as Jane Fonda and Raquel Welch. Barcelona native and Compar president Dr. Fernando Aleu brought together the magic of Paco Rabanne and the Puig family fragrance company for the creation of Calandre, blended by perfumer Michael Hy. The fragrance is a floral blend with cool greens and mossy woods; fresh, clean, and casual. When it was introduced, it was a shocking departure from the heavy, sweet, sensual fragrances of the past ushering in a new age of fresh, natural scents.

Calandre is French for "the grille of a car" and is intended to signify the modern woman's mobility. Rabanne explains: "Women today are on the move, traveling near and far to pursue careers of every endeavor. What could be a better symbol of this than the grille of a car?" Of a Ford Model-T, to be exact. This theme is carried through to the bottle, a sleek, modern design of glass and chrome from the talented team of Paco Rabanne and Pierre Dinand. The bottle is a stylized rendition of the grille and the New York United Nations building, selected to symbolize international appeal and cooperation.

Calandre has also undergone a reorchestration. Green notes accent a heart of predominately rose, and a sharp metallic edge lines the composition, creating a sleek, even more modern version of the original.

Jan's Note: You'll find similarities between Rive Gauche and Calandre which were produced within a year of each other. Rive Gauche was brought forth in 1970 and was a more complex, refined version of Calandre which is a leaner composition. As everything changes, the two fragrances are farther apart now with mutual reorchestrations, but still, similarities remain. Many aficionados wear both, though most are more ardent in their passion for one over the other. And so, the competition continues…

Scent Type: Powdery Floral
Top Notes: Greens, aldehydes, bergamot
Heart Notes: Rose, jasmine, lily of the valley, geranium, orris
Base Notes: Sandalwoods, vetiver, oakmoss, amber, musk

Who's Worn It
Lauren Bacall, Barbara Bush

Introduced: 1969

***

Calèche

Hermès

Calèche is a classic floral aldehyde, or powdery floral perfume, from Hermès. Created by master perfumer Guy Robert, Calèche is, quite simply, a remarkable masterpiece. A brilliant aldehydic opening adds verve and vivacity to a feminine floral heart of jasmine, gardenia, rose, and iris. A soft wooded finish completes the lovely, timeless arrangement. Calèche is the embodiment of the perfect spring day.

Calèche is housed in a clear glass flacon of simple elegance and wrapped with a yellow silk bow. It is presented in a vibrant spring yellow box embellished with the proud gold-colored symbol of the House of Hermès, a stately horse-drawn carriage, or *calèche*, which was the most elegant of

Vintage Perfumes

nineteenth-century carriages.

Jan's Note: Although the original formula seems to have undergone a renovation, Calèche remains a lovely statement, though perhaps a bit more suited to modern tastes.

Scent Type: Powdery Floral
Top Notes: Bergamot, lemon, aldehydes, neroli
Heart Notes: Gardenia, ylang-ylang, jasmine, rose, iris
Base Notes: Sandalwood, oakmoss, cedarwood, vetiver, amber, musk

Who's Worn It
Dame Elizabeth Taylor, Sandra Howard, Sandra Bernhardt

Introduced: 1961

***

Capricci
Nina Ricci

Cheerful. Seductive. Mesmerizing. Capricci charms with sensual flair. The classic floral bouquet hails from the firm established by French couturier Nina Ricci and her son, Robert Ricci, who oversaw fragrance development. He once said, "My aim is to dress reality in the color of dreams."

Brimming with rose and jasmine, the lively bouquet is brightened with the green freshness of hyacinth and leaves.

Gardenia, ylang-ylang, and lily of the valley form a white floral refrain which is warmed with musk and sandalwood. Indulge the romantic in you with Capricci. Created by perfumer Francis Fabron.

Scent Type: Classic Floral
Top Notes: Hyacinth, green leaves
Heart Notes: Jasmine, lily of the valley, rose, ylang-ylang, gardenia
Base Notes: Musk, sandalwood

Introduced: 1961

***

Chaldée
Jean Patou

Chaldée (pronounced Kal-day) is a 1927 Jean Patou fragrance that derives its name from the country of Sumer in ancient Babylonia where beautiful golden-skinned women once lived. Modern bathing suits made their first appearance as summer vacations to beachside resorts became the rage among young people.

Inspired by the new outdoor sports of the 1920s, tennis and swimming, French couturier Patou designed Chaldée so that the richness of florals and amber would be amplified by the sun's warmth.

Originally, Huile de Chaldée was the first ever suntan

Vintage Perfumes

lotion, but the scent proved so popular that Patou made a fragrance to match. Sporty women at Deauville and the Riviera embraced it, and Chaldée became a signature fragrance of the 1920s sports-minded aristocracy.

Jan's Note: Tastes and styles change through the years, and what was once considered a sporty perfume would now be considered too rich to wear under warm rays of the sun, having been replaced by brisk citrus and sheer aquatic scents. Nevertheless, Chaldée is still a fragrance that harkens to a holiday frame of mind.

Scent Type: Vanilla-Amber Oriental
Top Notes: Hyacinth, orange blossom
Heart Notes: Jasmine, narcissus
Base Notes: Opoponax, spices

Who's Worn It
Tennis star Suzanne Lenglen

Introduced: 1927

***

Chamade
Guerlain

Every Guerlain perfume has a story, and Chamade is true to course, inspired by renowned works in art and literature. Fifth-generation perfumer Jean-Paul Guerlain formulated this modern classic for the contemporary woman, the bewitching woman of strength, confidence, and liberation. Chamade features green top notes, a spicy floral heart, and an Oriental base of soft woods.

Chamade was created in 1969, partly inspired by Françoise Sagan's novel of the same name. Chamade has dual meaning in French: "the drumbeat of surrender" and "the wild beating of the heart." And according to our dictionary, chamade is a trumpet or drum signal sounded for retreat or parley, discussion, or truce. The bottle resembles an upside-down heart and was supposedly inspired by a woman who turned hearts upside down.

Chamade features a memorable note of crisp green hyacinth, along with a cassis-accented jasmine-rose bouquet, and a vanilla-sweetened finish. Elegant and smooth, Chamade is a versatile, easy-to-wear scent with a subtle yet tenacious powdery sillage.

The long-lived House of Guerlain has created memorable scents that reflect the nature and mood of their times. Guerlain has endured from the Romantic period of the 1800s, through the Napoléonic Empire, the Third Republic,

Vintage Perfumes

La Belle Époque, World War I, and the Roaring Twenties. During World War II, the factory was twice bombed and abandoned. Guerlain overcame adversity to rebuild and prosper and remain current with changing styles. Guerlain suggests Chamade for "an audacious and radiant woman...feminine, seductive, dynamic, and sensual."

Jan's Note: If ever there was a pearls-and-little-black-dress fragrance, Chamade is it. I can even sense a note of buttery soft gloves, a subtle leathery note I used to smell in my grandmother's glove drawer. The green hyacinth note is fresh and charming while the powdery floral heart is pure luxury. Refined and well-mannered, a definite five-star perfume.

Scent Type: Floral Oriental
Top Notes: Greens, galbanum, bergamot, hyacinth, aldehydes
Heart Notes: Rose, jasmine, lilac, clove
Base Notes: Vanilla, amber, benzoin, sandalwood, vetiver

Who's Worn It
Princess Grace of Monaco, Audrey Hepburn, Catherine Deneuve, Phyllis Diller, Glenn Close

Introduced: 1969

***

Chanel No. 5
Chanel

Chanel No. 5 was the first fragrance from Parisian couturier Gabrielle "Coco" Chanel, who was one of the first designers to introduce a perfume. According to Chanel, the secret behind Chanel No. 5 is an extraordinary blend of aldehydes—ingredients that defy categorization—combined with rich floral and warm ambery wooded notes. The effect forms a halo of scent, an inner glow, or incandescence, which is utterly lovely.

Smoothly proportioned, this classic fragrance with an effervescent personality is versatile enough to be worn for a variety of occasions, winter through summer. Or take a tip from Marilyn Monroe: When the press once asked what nightwear she wore to bed, she smiled and answered, "Chanel No. 5."

With a reputation as one of the world's most sophisticated, elegant fragrances, Chanel No. 5 has been known for years as the epitome of luxury in keeping with Chanel's fashion vision of simple elegance.

As for the name, Chanel once reported that when she asked perfumer Ernest Beaux to create a fragrance for her, he presented her with several scents, and she selected the bottle numbered "5." Coincidentally, her couture collection was scheduled for presentation on the fifth day of the fifth month: May 5th. Interpreting this as a good omen, she bestowed

Vintage Perfumes

upon the fragrance the name of Chanel No. 5 and placed it in a sleekly modern bottle.

And so, Chanel entered the fragrance industry. Indeed, it was the popularity of the early Chanel fragrances that spawned the designer fragrance industry of today.

And the flacon? Pure and minimal with pared-down polish in classic rectangular Chanel bottles. As the company states, "True elegance stems from subtlety."

Jan's Note: Chanel No. 5 has a distinct powdery signature—everyone will know what you're wearing. Even today I spritz the powdery perfume on my bed from time to time just to revel in this aromatic gem that's polished to perfection. Pure, multifaceted, unerringly chic—Chanel No. 5 is grace under pressure.

Some vintage perfumes have been edited over time due to lack of ingredient availability, government regulations, or cost, but over the years Chanel has strictly adhered to excellence, going so far as to own the rose and jasmine fields so that they always exercise control over the ingredients. They also employ their own perfumer, rather than depending on an oil house as most companies do, with the rare exception. This fanaticism for perfection in today's marketplace is nearly unparalleled. The result? The Chanel No. 5 of today remains amazingly true to the original 1922 composition which has maintained its brilliance nearly a century later.

Does all this mean it's right for you? Only you can be

the judge of that. As an old saying goes, "when the student is ready, the teacher appears."

Scent Type: Powdery Floral
Top Notes: Aldehydes, Grasse jasmine
Heart Notes: Rose, ylang-ylang, iris
Base Notes: Amber, patchouli

Who's Worn It
Emily Deschanel, Kate Moss, Katie Price, Celine Dion, Nicole Kidman, Catherine Deneuve, Marilyn Monroe, Andrea Marcovicci, Carole Bouquet

Introduced: 1921

***

Chanel No. 18
Chanel

A Les Exclusifs de Chanel classic fragrance, No. 18 is named after Chanel's Place Vendôme jewelry address and in recognition of the designer's first jewelry collection from 1932.

The silky floral fragrance earns its place in Chanel's perfume collection with the use of the coveted South American ambrette seed which is derived from equatorial hibiscus blossoms. Musty and sensual, the natural ingredient is a scarce, precious commodity. Soft as cashmere, the

Vintage Perfumes

beguiling No. 18 warms to the bloom of delicate rose with a powdery touch of iris.

No. 18 is a rare jewel for women who enjoy discreet, high quality collectibles. Blended by Jacques Polge and Christopher Sheldrake.

Jan's Note: Though Chanel No. 18 is one of the more recent vintage perfumes, it was included because of the vintage inspiration and its decidedly vintage feel. If you're sampling other vintage Chanel perfumes, this is certainly one to consider.

Scent Type: Floral – Rose-Iris
Top Notes: Hibiscus
Heart Notes: Rose, iris
Base Notes: Ambrette seed

Introduced: 1997

***

Chanel No. 19
Chanel

Chanel No. 19 was Coco Chanel's personal fragrance, said to have been named, partly, after her birth date of August 19. The fragrance opens with fresh green floral notes tempered with fragrant mosses and aromatic woods. Chanel No. 19 is a spare, spirited scent. Created for Mademoiselle when she was in her eighties by master perfumer Guy Robert, No. 19 is a starkly modern fragrance in keeping with her fashion vision.

Chanel's designs changed women's fashion forever. From humble beginnings, she founded her first store in Deauville, France in 1912 and went on to stamp her style throughout the twenties and thirties with the little black dress, bobbed haircuts, and a profusion of oversize costume jewelry.

She closed her operation when World War II broke out. After a long hiatus, the House of Chanel opened its doors again in 1954, and at the age of 71 she introduced the straight collarless suit that today is synonymous with Chanel.

Coco Chanel's life and romantic liaisons were as remarkable as her designs. She lived to see her life chronicled in a 1969 Broadway musical, *Coco*.

The Chanel company describes the slightly arrogant Chanel No. 19 in terms that were also applicable to Mademoiselle Chanel, as she was known, who died in 1971: "Forever young, intensely feminine, contemporary, brilliant, witty, outspoken, supremely confident, and completely independent." A lovely, lasting tribute to one of the world's most memorable women.

Or, as Mme Chanel once said, "In perfume, as in fashion, simple understatement is pure elegance."

Vintage Perfumes

Jan's Note: The Chanel numbered perfumes are interesting juxtapositions in artistry. Of all the Chanel perfumes, No. 19 is the one that reminds me most of Mme Chanel. Spare, arrogant, confident—and enormously talented. This is the least romanticized formula in the Chanel collection. No. 19 is a fragrance for women who mean business, but do it with enormous style.

Scent Type: Floral – Green
Top Notes: Greens, galbanum, bergamot
Heart Notes: Jasmine, may rose, iris, ylang-ylang
Base Notes: Sandalwood, oakmoss, vetiver

Who's Worn It
Catherine Deneuve, Christie Brinkley

Introduced: 1972

***

Chanel No. 22
Chanel

Gabrielle "Coco" Chanel designed Chanel No. 22, a mélange of white flowers, to shimmer like Champagne bubbles, a small ray of light as the world sank toward the darkness of the Depression. The floral symphony complemented her couture line known as the White Look, designs that celebrated the resurgence of joy, romance, and femininity.

Interestingly, perfume No. 22 is one of the perfume samples that perfumer Ernest Beaux presented to Mme Chanel when she was making a selection for the fragrance that became known as No. 5.

In this powdery floral, roses, jasmine, and orange blossoms dominate with a profusion of white flowers. No. 22 is a sweet blend of florals—soft, satiny, and sensuous. Decidedly feminine with a bright aldehydic rush. Pure vintage.

Jan's Note: Chanel's No. 5 and No. 22 are both aldehydic floral perfumes, though No. 22 features a bounty of white flowers and iris along with the vivid sharp sparkle of aldehydes that both formulas share. If you've worn No. 5 for a long time and are looking for something different, yet fundamentally similar, try No. 22.

Scent Type: Powdery Floral
Notes: White roses, jasmine, tuberose, iris, lily of the valley, lilac, orange blossom

Who's Worn It
Catherine Deneuve, Isabel Toledo

Introduced: 1928

***

Vintage Perfumes

Chant d'Arômes
Guerlain

Chant d'Arômes, meaning "song of scent" in French, is a light, playful scent designed by Jean-Paul Guerlain. The company says it was created "for the debutantes of life as a first perfume."

A powdery floral, peachy chypre fragrance, it was partly inspired by poet Saint-John Perse, who "dreamed of an isle greener than dreams." Guerlain imagined the aromas that might be found on such an idyllic island, and the result was Chant d'Arômes, a fragrance of innocence and tenderness, a scent of eternal youth.

True to his vision, Chant d'Arômes opens with island-fresh fruits, followed by a spicy floral heart and sweet balsamic background notes tinged with fresh moss. Soft, discreet, refined.

The House of Guerlain was a court-appointed perfumer to many of the royal courts of Europe. From Queen Victoria of England to Empress Eugénie of France, Queen Isabella of Spain to Empress Sissi of Austria, Guerlain fragrances have graced the world's most fashionable and influential women of the last two centuries, as well as those of today. Even the unforgettable Sarah Bernhardt commissioned her own Guerlain scent during the height of La Belle Époque.

Jan's Note: Sweet, soft, innocent. Chant d'Arômes was Jean-Paul Guerlain's first perfume after taking over from his father, Jacques Guerlain. His youthful outlook is apparent in this charming, effervescent perfume, though his skill and training is clearly on display and only improved with age. Utterly lovely.

Scent Type: Chypre – Floral
Top Notes: Mirabelle peach, gardenia, aldehydes, fruits
Heart Notes: Rose, jasmine, honeysuckle, ylang-ylang
Base Notes: Benzoin, musk, vetiver, heliotrope, moss, olibanum

Who's Worn It
Lynn Redgrave, Shirley Bassey

Introduced: 1962

***

Chantilly
Houbigant

Chantilly is a classic French blend of florals, Oriental woods, and spices with a sweet amber finish. An expansive fragrance originally created by Houbigant, Chantilly enchants with a heart of jasmine and rose, smoothed with vanilla, musk, and tonka bean.

Chantilly shares its name with the picturesque French

Vintage Perfumes

town, the pastoral site of championship Thoroughbred horse racing. Perfect for a day at the races with a broad-brimmed hat and dark sunglasses just as your grandmother might have once enjoyed when she was young.

Jan's Note: Chantilly is one of the vintage perfumes that has undergone revisions. Though somewhat removed from its original splendor, it remains a simple, nostalgic pleasure.

Scent Type: Oriental – Vanilla Ambery
Top Notes: Fruits, lemon, bergamot, neroli
Heart Notes: Jasmine, rose, orange blossom, spices, ylang-ylang, carnation
Base Notes: Indian sandalwood, moss, vanilla, musk, leather, tonka bean, benzoin

Introduced: 1941

***

Cinnabar
Estée Lauder

Cinnabar is a spicy Oriental fragrance from Estée Lauder. Opening citrus notes add a fresh lift to the sultry, exotic scent.

Revel in the mystery of Cinnabar. Tangerine adds a fresh lift to the exotic elixir while sultry sandalwood, clove, and patchouli warm a magnetic heart of lily and rose. Sensual and surreal, the balsamic Cinnabar is reminiscent of Far Eastern aromas and visions of ancient luxury.

Under the early stewardship of founder Estée Lauder, legend has it that she personally added the final ingredients to guarded perfume formulas to ensure secrecy. One whiff of the balsamic Cinnabar potion and you can just imagine Lauder meticulously measuring those last drops.

Jan's Note: Cinnabar devotees are a quiet army of admirers. This spicy Oriental blend is a 1978 classic, when perfumes were big and bold and audacious. From Giorgio to Opium, these fragrances reflected a time when women were asserting their independence. Cinnabar is a well-priced fragrance in the same family as Opium or Must de Cartier. Definitely worth a try.

Scent Type: Spicy-Woody Oriental
Top Notes: Jasmine, orange blossom, tangerine
Heart Notes: Lily, lily of the valley, clove
Base Notes: Patchouli, sandalwood, olibanum

Introduced: 1978

***

Vintage Perfumes

Citrus Bigarrade
Creed

A classic dry citrus eau de cologne from Creed, Citrus Bigarrade (meaning "dry citrus" in French) was originally blended for Edward, Duke of Windsor. Legend has it that the Duchess wore it, too.

After the initial crisp citrus, a soft, spritely green heart of neroli emerges, anchored with the smooth finish of ambergris.

From 1946, Citrus Bigarrade is a fragrance fit for the man who gave up his throne for the stylish American woman with whom he spent the remainder of his years traveling the globe in the height of style.

Scent Type: Citrus
Top Notes: Bergamot, citrus notes
Heart Notes: Neroli, orange blossom
Base Notes: Ambergris

Who's Worn It
The Duke and Duchess of Windsor, Douglas Fairbanks

Introduced: 1946
***

JAN MORAN

Climat
Lancôme

From 1967, Climat is a smooth floral fragrance created by perfumer Gerard Goupy for the French firm of Lancôme. Climat begins with brisk essences of violet, bergamot, and peach that flow into an elegant heart of lily of the valley, jasmine, and rose. A subtle, ambery-wooded base provides a quietly sensual and soothing finale.

Elegant and endearing, Climat is a fragrance of classic proportion, a versatile, multifaceted scent for the woman with a certain indefinable something, a certain *je ne sais quoi*. Climat is perfume of sophistication and individuality.

Jan's Note: Slightly restructured but still lovely. Climat is a young Parisienne, a breath of spring, a perfume of infinite possibilities.

Scent Type: Green Floral
Top Notes: Peach, bergamot, violet
Heart Notes: Heliotrope, jasmine, lily of the valley, narcissus, rose
Base Notes: Sandalwood, vetiver, amber

Introduced: 1967

***

Vintage Perfumes

Cocktail

Jean Patou

Cocktail is a witty, refreshing splash of citrus fruits and oakmoss, a classic chypre combination. Created in 1930 by French couturier Jean Patou, it was inspired by the art of original mixing. Crisp and easy to wear, day through evening, Cocktail is a glamorous retro scent enjoying a new lease on life. It's a clever scent to wear with your little black cocktail dress. Anyone for a martini or cosmopolitan?

In the 1930s, Patou provided a burl and glass cocktail bar in his salon to amuse the gentlemen while the women were being fitted. Along with the usual libations, an assortment of essential oils was also available to patrons so that they could create their own fragrances.

The array of classic Patou fragrances takes us back to this ingenious cocktail bar tradition, reminding us of the excesses of the twenties, of the flamboyant jazz age, of aristocratic summers at the Riviera and Deauville, and of the racy Hispano Suiza automobile Patou motored throughout Europe.

Jan's Note: Cheers! Need I say more?

Scent Type: Chypre – Fruity
Top Notes: Greens, bergamot, citrus
Heart Notes: Jasmine, rose
Base Notes: Oakmoss

Who's Worn It
Vivian Leigh

Introduced: 1930

***

Coco
Chanel

Coco was created in honor of couturier Gabrielle Chanel. Colleagues called her "Mademoiselle," but her dearest friends knew her as "Coco." The scent that bears the affectionate nickname is said to embody "the spirit of Chanel…a microcosm of youth, desire, daring, sensuality, force, and fragility."

A warm spicy fragrance, Coco develops around a major amber chord. Mellow fruits, heady florals, and exotic spices are balanced against woods and leathers, creating a rich, smooth balsamic blend. Artfully composed, Coco is a fragrance of sensuality and glamour.

The perfume comes in the familiar rectangular flacon favored by Chanel, while other strengths are sold in sleek black and gold-colored lacquered bottles that travel well.

Vintage Perfumes

As Coco Chanel once said, "Elegance is not possible without fragrance."

Jan's Note: Coco manages to balance sensuality and refined good taste. While dramatic, it's not too over-the-top. The leathery note adds an earthy smokiness to spicy mélange. A beautiful perfume for autumn and winter. If you enjoy spicy floral Orientals, Coco is not to be missed. Although Coco is one of the more recent vintages, it has definitely earned its place among the finest legendary perfumes.

Scent Type: Floral Oriental
Top Notes: Peach, Comoros Island orange blossom, coriander
Heart Notes: Spice Island clove bud, Caribbean cascarida, French angelica, Bulgarian rose, Indian jasmine, mimosa, frangipani
Base Notes: Mysore sandalwood, amber, leather

Who's Worn It
Gwyneth Paltrow, Vanessa Paradis, Catherine Zeta-Jones

Introduced: 1984
***

JAN MORAN

Cœur Joie (Coeur Joie)
Nina Ricci

Parisian artistry. Vintage charm. Coeur Joie, meaning "joyful heart," is a radiant floral bouquet from French couturier Nina Ricci who was known for graceful, romantic designs. From 1946, Coeur Joie was her debut fragrance, developed with perfumer Germaine Cellier, one of the few female perfumers of her time.

Evocative as an Impressionist painting: Soft, velvety iris blooms amidst a lacy garland of gardenia, rose, and jasmine. Hyacinth adds an unexpected sparkle of verdant green brilliance. Aldehydes—powdery and elegant—gild Coeur Joie with pure romance. An elusive sillage of amber and musk warms to the skin like the glow of golden sunshine.

The charming heart-shaped bottle, a coveted collector's item, was a collaboration of artist Christian Berard, Marc Lalique, and Ricci's son, Robert Ricci, who oversaw Nina Ricci perfumes. He once said of Coeur Joie, which was created after the end of World War II, "I wanted [Coeur Joie] to be noble and cheerful, reflecting the joy of victory, freedom, and happiness found again!"

Jan's Note: From packing to perfume, Coeur Joie remains the essence of romance. A spring-fresh floral with powdery iris, the perfume can still be found as part of a prestige collection on the Nina Ricci website.

Vintage Perfumes

Scent Type: Powdery Floral
Top Notes: Hyacinth, aldehydes
Heart Notes: Iris, jasmine, rose, gardenia
Base Notes: Musk, amber

Introduced: 1946

***

Colony
Jean Patou

In 1938, debonair French couturier Jean Patou introduced Colony, a fragrance inspired by early French colonial holdings with sun-drenched ports, lush vegetation, exotic spices, and tropical sands. Imagine Catherine Deneuve in the film classic, Indochine.

Voluptuous fruits and jungle flowers are combined with woods and leathery notes to produce a chypre composition. Such blends are characterized by the marriage of fresh citrus and velvety moss and are also known as mossy-woody blends.

In the 1930s and 1940s, Colony was a favorite bon-voyage gift for many a high sea journey. Why not reminisce and pack the retro-glamour Colony for your next summer cruise?

Jan's Note: Colony captures the spirit of the late 1930s, in the era between the Great Depression and World War II. To wear Colony is to venture into the past.

Scent Type: Chypre - Fruity
Top Notes: Pineapple, bergamot
Heart Notes: Ylang-ylang, iris, carnation, opopanax
Base Notes: Oakmoss, leather, musk, vetiver, vanilla

Introduced: 1938

***

Cristalle
Chanel

Cristalle begins as a crisp citrus scent that segues into a deeper fruity chypre blend. A classic perfume from Chanel, it was originally developed as a single-strength eau de toilette to be lavished all over the body. In addition to the eau de toilette, a new strength was introduced in 1993, a richer eau de parfum version with a few changes.

"A respect for one's roots and an attachment to the origins of Cristalle were the foundation of the new scent," said Jacques Polge, perfumer and director of the Chanel Perfume Laboratories.

The eau de toilette version of Cristalle is a light energetic scent with a tangy top note of lemon, more citrus, and brighter green herbal notes. The eau de parfum is a richer composition with a few twists. Fruity mandarin replaces zesty lemon, jasmine is emphasized while greens and herbs are de-emphasized, mellow lily of the valley is added, and iris and woods are increased for new warmth and depth.

Both versions are dynamic fragrances that remind us of Mademoiselle Chanel, whose unconstructed clothing designs were suitable for sporting activities which was a radical concept in the early part of the century. Fresh and spirited, Cristalle is easy elegance.

Scent Type: Citrus – Chypre
Top Notes: Greens, mandarin, lemon, bergamot, galbanum, basil, lavender
Heart Notes: Rose, hyacinth, honeysuckle, jasmine, peach, lily of the valley, ylang-ylang, iris, mosses
Base Notes: Woods, musk, fruits, sandalwood, oakmoss

Who's Worn It
Rachel Weisz, Claudia Schiffer, Juliette Binoche

Introduced: 1977
***

Cuir de Russie
Chanel

Vintage haute parfumerie. Cuir de Russie Chanel is a reintroduction of Gabrielle Chanel's elegant 1927 fragrance, a perfume reminiscent of a glamorous bygone era. Mademoiselle Chanel, or "Coco" to her friends, created Cuir de Russie in what is known as her Russian period, during which her deep friendship with a Russian prince inspired her couture collections. Introduced in conjunction with two other scents, Gardénia and Bois des Îles, Cuir de Russie is reminiscent of a glamorous bygone era.

Cuir de Russie, or "Russian leather," is a vibrant leathery, woody composition by master perfumer Ernest Beaux. A floral bouquet of orange blossom, rose, and jasmine adds understated elegance. An inviting classic, Cuir de Russie is the perfect accent for a special evening at New York's legendary Russian Tea Room restaurant, or anytime you want to warm a winter's eve.

Jan's Note: To me, Cuir de Russie is cognac on a winter's eve at the Paris Ritz, après-ski in Aspen, a sleigh ride in Switzerland. Warm, tactile, and opulent. Vintage glamour, bottled.

Vintage Perfumes

Scent Type: Chypre – Leather
Top Notes: Styrax, birch, orange blossom, bergamot, mandarin, clary sage
Heart Notes: Iris, jasmine, rose, ylang-ylang, cedarwood, vetiver
Base Notes: Balsamics, leather, amber, vanilla

Introduced: 1927

***

Diorama

Dior

In 1949, perfumer Edmond Roudnitska created Diorama, the second fragrance after Miss Dior. In this exotic, cumin-laced white floral affair, Roudnitska's masterful touch was clearly evident.

More than fifty years later in a new century, perfumer François Demachy oversaw the reorchestration of Diorama. Ylang-ylang and jasmine form the white floral bouquet while patchouli leads the finale. A spicy note of dry cumin is evident throughout, which was the genius of Roudnitska.

A once rare collectible among vintage perfume connoisseurs and collectors, Diorama has returned in all its vintage glamour and sophistication.

Jan's Note: A must-have for avid Dior fashion collectors.

Scent Type: Chypre - Floral
Top Notes: Ylang-ylang, bergamot, peach, plum
Heart Notes: Egyptian cumin, Turkish rose, Indian jasmine
Base Notes: Indonesian patchouli, cedarwood

Introduced: 1949

***

Diorella
Dior

Diorella is an ethereal chypre blend from Christian Dior. Blended by legendary perfumer Edmond Roudnitska, the perfume combines sheer sunlit warmth with startling tenacity. A scent of verve and vitality, Diorella splashes on with cool lemon and basil followed by radiant honeysuckle and jasmine. An earthy-mossy base is blended of woody vetiver and oakmoss.

The fragrance is a superb example of the classic citrus-moss chypre blend, so named after the Mediterranean island of Cyprus where many of the ingredients are found.

Christian Dior apprenticed in Paris at the atelier of Robert Piguet before opening his own salon in 1946. His timing was perfect, and his feminine New Look collection of swirling skirts, tiny waists, and glamorous gowns became the rage in postwar Paris. Dior's classic suits set the trend in the fifties until his death in 1957. The reins then passed to a twenty-one-year-old named Yves Saint Laurent, who headed the company until 1960 when he left to serve in the Algerian war. Today the House of Dior still leads the way with artful creations in fashion and fragrance.

Enjoy a slice of history with the radiant, sunshine-citrus blend that is the heart of Diorella.

Jan's Note: Diorella has been refurbished for government compliance but still retains the marvelous creative signature of Roudnitska, a master of perfumery. For those who love the masculine Eau Savage, Diorella is the feminine answer. Actually, I love to wear Eau Savage myself, and many men might enjoy wearing Diorella. True art knows no gender. Yes, Roudnitska was that talented.

Scent Type: Chypre – Fresh
Top Notes: Sicilian lemon, greens, basil, Italian bergamot, melon
Heart Notes: Moroccan jasmine, rose, carnation, cyclamen
Base Notes: Oakmoss, vetiver, musk, patchouli

Introduced: 1972

***

JAN MORAN

Dioressence
Dior

Dioressence is a sophisticated Oriental blend of florals and spices from Christian Dior, a voluptuous, opulent fragrance for women of style and confidence. Dioressence is beautiful for cool symphony evenings under a layer of cashmere.

Since its initial incarnation in 1969 by perfumers Guy Robert and Max Gavarry, Dioressence has undergone a transformation. Vetiver and oakmoss (blended to resemble oakmoss, that is) add an earthy green backlight to this spiced floral composition.

Jan's Note: If you haven't tried Dioressnce in a long time, try it again. The formula has been finely edited and modernized. A breeze of green freshness adds a chypre note to the Oriental blend now. Dioressence is one of five original Dior perfumes overseen by Christian Dior (along with Diorama, Diorling, Diorella, and Diorissimo) which he had created to launch alongside his fashion collection. He affectionately referred to these as 'dresses in a bottle,' meaning these perfumes captured the essence of his designs.

Vintage Perfumes

Scent Type: Spicy-Woody Oriental
Top Notes: Aldehydes, greens, fruits
Heart Notes: Jasmine, geranium, cinnamon, carnation, tuberose, ylang-ylang, orris
Base Notes: Patchouli, oakmoss, vetiver, benzoin, vanilla, musk, styrax

Introduced: 1969

***

Diorissimo
Dior

Diorissimo is the perfumer's interpretation of lily of the valley which refuses to yield its essence, so it must be recreated for perfumery from the perfumer's palette. Master perfumer Edmond Roudnitska achieved the near impossible of recreating nature in this excellent rendition.

In Diorissimo, the dominant note is the light, ethereal essence of lily of the valley which couturier Christian Dior considered his lucky flower and Roudnitska grew in his garden. In fact, Dior tucked a sprig of lily of the valley for luck into every creation that ventured onto the runway. In perfumer's terms, this "stylized" lily of the valley bouquet remains the most personal of Dior's many fragrances.

Roudnitska, who is said to have relied upon dreamlike springtime images to create Diorissimo, once described Diorissimo, saying, "This is a pure lily of the valley scent that also has the odor of the woods in which it is found and the indefinable atmosphere of springtime."

Thus the airy, celestial quality of the fragrance. Always right, never overpowering. Diorissimo is a delicate floral, very feminine, fresh, innocent, and romantic.

Jan's Note: While reformulated for governmental compliance, Diorissimo retains its vintage charm.

Scent Type: Floral – Fresh
Top Notes: Greens, bergamot, calyx
Heart Notes: Lily of the valley, jasmine, boronia, rosewood, ylang-ylang, lilac
Base Notes: Sandalwood, civet

Who's Worn It
Naomi Campbell, Amanda Harlech, Diana, Princess of Wales, Amy Astley

Introduced: 1956
***

Diorling
Dior

A dark, leathery floral from 1963, Diorling was a demanding mistress of perfumery. The modern recreation is toned down, more politically correct, but still a lovely floral with a leathery finish.

The brilliance of jasmine serves as a foil to the leathery patchouli accord, and the finale is fresher and more modern than the original. Vintage Diorling was nearly impossible to find and hoarded by collectors. The modern Diorling is still reminiscent of the original, though in a lighter, contemporary manner.

Scent Type: Chypre – Floral/Leather
Top Notes: Bergamot
Heart Notes: Jasmine
Base Notes: Patchouli, leather accord

Introduced: 1963

***

Eau d'Hadrien
Annick Goutal

Eau d'Hadrien is a refreshing, refined citrus fragrance that can be worn by women and men. The understated scent from Annick Goutal is generally offered in a light eau de toilette, as well as a more concentrated eau de parfum. Lemon, grapefruit, and citron form a traditional-style eau de cologne accord with a green wooded finish of cypress.

Eau d'Hadrien was Goutal's personal morning scent; the fresh fragrance she splashed on and wore at home in the early hours. As the day progressed, she recommended layering other fragrances from her collection right over it. In fact, the entire Goutal line is made to be mixed and layered for unique interpretations.

Jan's Note: Eau d'Hadrien is a wonderful fragrance in the Annick Goutal line. It's a smooth, refined citrus fragrance, ideal for those who dislike sharp citrus scents. If you have other Annick Goutal perfumes such as Rose Absolue, Passion, or Gardénia Passion, try adding a spritz of Eau d'Hadrien as a top layer. The fresh citrus notes and warm wooded finish will add new dimensions to floral and ambery Oriental fragrances. This is ideal in spring and summer when you wish to add a fresher element to your rich winter fragrances.

Scent Type: Chypre - Fresh (unisex)
Notes: Sicilian lemon, grapefruit, citron, cypress

Who's Worn It
Nicole Kidman, Celine Dion, Liv Tyler, Oprah, Steven Spielberg, Prince, Madonna, Tina Turner, Leonardo Di Caprio, Prince Charles, Queen Noor, Samantha Boardman, Catherine Deneuve, Tom Cruise

Introduced: 1986
***

Vintage Perfumes

Eau d'Hermès
Hermès

Eau d'Hermès is a noble unisex fragrance created by master perfumer Edward Roudnitska. A celestial blend of citrus, spice, and florals, it is subtly enhanced with a touch of woods. It was relaunched on the 150th anniversary of the House of Hermès. Another classic fragrance from Hermès Paris, Eau de Hermès is a fresh, invigorating blend suitable for both men and women. Wear it for daytime, summer, or anytime a fresh scent is preferred. Perhaps right after a sunrise canter on your trusty horse with the Hermès saddle, your favorite silk Hermès scarf soaring in the breeze behind you. Ah...we live for luxuries.

Scent Type: Citrus
Top Notes: Cardamom, herbal lavender, petitgrain lemon, cinnamon, cumin
Heart Notes: Jasmine, Bourbon geranium, vanilla, tonka bean, labdanum
Base Notes: Sandalwood, cedarwood, flamed birch

Who's Worn It
Angie Dickinson

Introduced: 1951

JAN MORAN

Eau d'Orange Verte
Hermès

Since 1837, the French house of Hermès has brought forth luxury goods of every description, from the finest leathers and silks to the most exquisite fragrances.

A scent for men and women, Eau d'Orange Verte from Hermès is a crisp, refreshing citrus blend. The inclusion of peppermint adds freshness and vigor, while sweet orange and mandarin are blended with petit grain lemon for a fruity-woody drydown.

Sporty and chic, Eau d'Orange Verte is housed in a tall green bottle. Perfect for steamy city days and beach-front evenings.

Scent Type: Citrus
Top Notes: Peppermint, mandarin
Heart Notes: Sweet orange
Base Notes: Petit grain lemon, orange tree leaves

Who's Worn It
Rainer Andreesen

Introduced: 1979

***

Vintage Perfumes

Eau de Camille
Annick Goutal

Eau de Camille was created by Renaissance woman Annick Goutal, a former concert pianist, model, and an accomplished perfumer.

This fragrance was named in honor of her daughter, Camille. One day her daughter opened a window in their home in France, and Goutal was inspired by the scents wafting through, the smell of ivy and vines and fresh-cut grass, of honeysuckle and other fresh florals. This crisp green floral is usually available in a light eau de toilette and a concentrated eau de parfum.

When Annick Goutal passed away in 1999, Camille took her mother's creative place in the company working with perfumer Isabelle Doyen on new creations.

Goutal once said of her creative endeavor: "Nature and all her wonders guide me. Emotions find expression in fragrance. Fragrance is the music of my dreams. Fragrance is my inspiration." A toast to a lovely, talented woman.

Jan's Note: For a true delight, visit the Goutal boutique on the rue de Castiglione in Paris' elegant Seventh Arrondissement. It's like walking into a fairyland of perfume.

Scent Type: Floral – Green
Notes: Honeysuckle, ivy, grass, seringa

Who's Worn It
Isabelle Adjani, Andrea Marcovicci

Introduced: 1986
***

Eau de Campagne
Sisley

Nature's bounty is mirrored in Eau de Campagne, a classic fragrance for women or men. From Sisley, the firm established by Count Hubert and Countess Isabelle d'Ornano, the revitalizing scent is awash in zesty meadow-fresh essences. Basil, lemon, galbanum, and lily of the valley form a spirited spring impression while patchouli, oakmoss, and vetiver create a rich mossy finish.

Eau de Campagne is the fragrance of country life, of rich soil, fresh air, and verdant fields. It's no wonder; Sisley specializes in natural beauty products based on the process of phytocosmetology, which is the use of botanical plant material.

Vintage Perfumes

Scent Type: Fougère
Top Notes: Herbs, lemon, basil, bergamot, galbanum
Heart Notes: Jasmine, lily of the valley, tomato leaves, geranium
Base Notes: Musk, oakmoss, vetiver

Introduced: 1974

***

Eau de Cologne
Chanel

Chanel perfumer Jacques Polge's Les Exclusifs de Chanel collection is an ode to the art of perfumery. His Eau de Cologne is an artistic rendition of Chanel's 1929 classic, a sparkling ray of light in a bucolic spring garden.

The vibrant citrus blend features lemon, petitgrain, and bergamot, but it is neroli—the elegant and sublimely seductive heart of the orange blossom—that lifts this Eau de Cologne to the high standards of Chanel. It's fresh and invigorating with a cashmere-soft sheen of musk. Eau de Cologne is ideal paired with any chic daytime ensemble—for women and men alike.

"As a creator of perfumes, I am dedicated to the search for a scent which responds to the needs and desires of women today, and helps them to achieve their own individuality." Jacques Polge, perfumer.

Jan's Note: If you're a connoisseur of eaux de cologne, add this to your list—unless, of course, you've already fallen head-over-heels in love with Chanel's elegant version of the classic eau de cologne.

Scent Type: Citrus
Notes: Lemon, neroli, petitgrain, bergamot

Introduced: 1929

***

Eau de Cologne du Coq
Guerlain

Eau de Cologne du Coq is a legendary creation from perfumer Jacques Guerlain. This century-old classic is a dry, crisp citrus splash with a lavender heart. Available only in cologne, it is packaged in the distinctive "bee bottle," a flacon created in honor of the Napoléonic court.

Eaux de cologne are often classified as "hesperides," meaning that they are made from the fruit of citrus trees. In Greek mythology, Hesperides were garden nymphs who guarded the wedding gift of golden apples from Gaea to Hera. Hesperia was also the ancient Greek name for Italy and the Roman name for Spain.

Most of these hesperides, or citrus eaux de cologne, are worn by any gender. Good for sporty active wear, hot humid days, or high-pressure offices.

Vintage Perfumes

Scent Type: Citrus
Top Notes: Hesperides, lemon, bergamot, neroli
Heart Notes: Lavender, jasmine, patchouli
Base Notes: Moss, sandalwood

Who's Worn It
Kirk Douglas

Introduced: 1894

***

Eau de Cologne Impériale
Guerlain

Eau de Cologne Impériale is a timeless, invigorating citrus scent that has been used by men and women for well over a century. The lime-citrus blend is lightened with orange blossom and minty rosemary. A stimulating, subtle blend, it can be worn anytime.

As the name suggests, Eau de Cologne Impériale is a fragrance of royalty. Master perfumer Pierre-François-Pascal Guerlain, the founder of the House of Guerlain, created the fragrance for the Empress Eugénie and placed it in a flacon known as the "bee bottle" to honor the Empire. The bee was a symbol of the Royal Court and of the industriousness of the Second Napoléonic Empire. Today, the French imperial crest is still prominently displayed on the bee bottle.

Empress Eugénie was born in Spain and became the wife

of the second Louis Napoléon, also known as Napoléon III. Noted for her beauty, she favored fragrances from the House of Guerlain and gowns from the House of Worth. Due to her patronage and enjoyment of fine fragrances, the House of Guerlain made rapid advances among its well-to-do clientele. Eau Impériale remains one of the most enduring fragrances of our time.

Scent Type: Citrus
Top Notes: Hesperides, orange blossom, bergamot, neroli, lemon
Heart Notes: Lavender, lime
Base Notes: Rosemary, tonka bean, cedarwood

Who's Worn It
Empress Eugénie, Cary Grant, Paul Newman, Marcello Mastrionni, Sir Alec Guiness, George Segal, President Ronald Reagan

Introduced: 1853

***

Vintage Perfumes

Eau de Guerlain
Guerlain

Eau de Guerlain is a fresh, sparkling *eau fraîche* composed by Jean-Paul Guerlain. It's a first-class eau de cologne formulation for both genders.

In eighteenth-century England, the Victorians assigned meaning to flowers, herbs, and plants. While some of these terms are merely romantic, others are quite fitting. For example, in the Victorian language of flowers, lemon blossoms signify zest and thyme is the symbol of activity, an appropriate description for this vigorous herb.

Eau de Guerlain has dominant notes of verbena flanked by lemon and thyme, mint and lavender. Fresh, clean, and stimulating, it's a perennial star in the Guerlain galaxy.

Jan's Note: Eau de Guerlain is one of the finest examples of eau de cologne. Verbena is one of my favorite scents, and Guerlain brings it forth beautifully in this composition.

Scent Type: Citrus
Top Notes: Lemon, bergamot, verbena, basil, petitgrain, fruits, caraway
Heart Notes: Neroli, thyme, mint, lavender, jasmine, carnation, rose
Base Notes: Tonka bean, forest moss, sandalwood

Who's Worn It
Bridget Fonda

Introduced: 1974

***

Eau de Patou
Jean Patou

From the French company of Jean Patou comes a crisp citrus scent meant to be liberally splashed on the skin. A crisp, refreshing eau de cologne that may be worn by women or men, it features top notes of orange and lime balanced by a fresh rose and honeysuckle heart. Subtle green moss, warm musk, and amber form a lingering impression on the skin.

Though a relatively new entry into the classic cologne hall of fame, Eau de Patou has nevertheless earned its rightful place. Packaged in ringed frosted glass flacons with sporty accents of marine blue and white.

Scent Type: Citrus
Top Notes: Sicilian citron, Guinea oranges, Grasse petitgrain
Heart Notes: Tunisian orange blossom, pepper, nasturtium, honeysuckle, ylang-ylang
Base Notes: Musk, moss, amber, civet, labdanum

Introduced: 1976

Vintage Perfumes

Eau Sauvage
Dior

Eau Sauvage is a robust citrus classic from Christian Dior. Elegant and ageless, the 1966 scent is a perennial favorite with gentlemen of distinction, and yet, women also embrace this quietly sensual scent.

Created by master perfumer Edmond Roudnitska, the fragrance opens with a lemon-rosemary zest bracing the senses for a green basil heart. Rich vetiver provides the perfect wooded foil to the citrus explosion. The refined drydown is a statement of quiet confidence.

Roudnitska was also the creative genius behind other classics, such as Diorella, Diorissimo, and Femme for Rochas. If one were to analyze these artistic achievements, the stylistic similarities are clear. In *Perfumes: The A to Z Guide*, authors Luca Turin and Tania Sanchez note the connection between Diorella and Eau Sauvage.

Excellence endures in Eau Sauvage.

Jan's Note: To me, Eau Sauvage is the scent of summer. It was also one of the first masculine fragrances I seized and claimed as my own. The rosemary note is fresh and earthy while the citrus notes capture the brilliance of the summer sun.

I once saw of photo of President Kennedy and Jacqueline aboard a boat—they were casually attired, enjoying a relaxing afternoon of just being Jack and Jackie, but even then, their elegance was unmistakable. Eau Sauvage is a fragrance much like that.

Scent Type: Aromatic Fougère
Top Notes: Bergamot, lemon, rosemary
Heart Notes: Lavender, Hedione
Base Notes: Vetiver

Who's Worn It
Claudia Schiffer, Antonio Banderas, Jude Law, Michael Douglas

Introduced: 1966
***

En Avion
Caron

It was 1932; Art Deco was in its stylish heyday and aviation in its thrilling infancy. Ernest Daltroff, founder of the French house of Caron, created En Avion in tribute to the daring women piloting the skies—and specifically, Amelia Earhart. A lusty, grand perfume, En Avion is born of courageous artistry.

The feminine floral Oriental is blended of opulent florals: jasmine, rose, and carnation. Orange lends its sunny disposition while an amber and wood base excites with fiery

Vintage Perfumes

exuberance. En Avion is an elegant fragrance for women who defy the odds. Savor it for wintry cashmere days and snowy silken evenings.

In 1904, perfumer Ernest Daltroff established the house of Caron in Paris. Renowned for his artistry, Daltroff created some of the world's most enchanting perfumes for women and men, including Narcisse Noir, Nuit de Noel, and Pour Homme. Today, under the guidance of a new owner, the house of Caron continues to produce Daltroff's vintage line along with new Caron creations.

Jan's Note: The reorchestration of En Avion brings forth the rose and citrus and lessens the spicy wooded notes in favor of modernization, sort of like a propeller plane that's been upgraded with a jet engine. Even so, the romance of early aviation still captures my imagination.

Scent Type: Floral Oriental
Top Notes: Orange
Heart Notes: Jasmine, rose
Base Notes: Amber, carnation

Who's Worn It
Isabelle Adjani

Introduced: 1932

***

Epicéa
Creed

Epicéa, meaning "spicy" in French, is a spicy woody fougère blend from Creed. Created in 1965, Epicéa is a well-balanced blend of refreshing bergamot, spicy-sweet clove, and Russian spruce wood.

Perfumer Olivier Creed, who was inspired by wintry countrysides and the warmth of a crackling fireplace, explains, "Epicéa evokes the élan of chalet life. Many say the fragrance calls to mind the joy of holidays in wintry climes, clear nights and starlight glistening on snow-covered hills."

Scent Type: Fougère – Spicy Woody
Notes: Lavender, clove, bergamot, spruce wood

Who's Worn It
Gary Cooper

Introduced: 1965

***

Estée
Estée Lauder

Estée Lauder's namesake fragrance is a rich floral composition for the confident woman. Raspberry enlivens sweet essences of jasmine, rose, and lily of the valley. The finale of powdery woods and sensual musk is tenacious, yet refined.

Versatile and sophisticated, Estée was created by perfumer Bernard Chant, a legend in perfumery. Estée captures the spirit and style of Estée Lauder, one of the world's most successful beauty experts, whose remarkable story began with a skin treatment formula that spawned her signature line of color cosmetics, skin care, and fragrance.

In terms of vintage perfumery, Estée reflects the conflicting social climate of 1968 with *Mad Men* styles and emerging women's rights issues.

Scent Type: Floral
Top Notes: Peach, raspberry, citrus oils
Heart Notes: Rose, lily of the valley, jasmine, carnation, ylang-ylang, honey, orris
Base Notes: Cedarwood, musk, moss, sandalwood, styrax

Who's Worn It
Nancy Reagan, Pat Buckly, Duchess of Windsor

Introduced: 1968

***

JAN MORAN

Fantasia de Fleurs
Creed

Spring is in the air. Fantasia de Fleurs is a rich floral fantasy from Creed. Abundant with the brilliance of sun-kissed flowers, from romantic rose to powdery iris, Fantasia de Fleurs is a tribute to femininity, vintage style.

Fantasia de Fleurs was created for Empress Elisabeth of Austria-Hungary, also known as Sisi, who was celebrated and emulated for her style and beauty. Legend has it that her elaborate chestnut coiffure was often perfumed with Fantasia de Fleurs.

Creed has long created masterpiece perfumes for royalty, dignitaries, and celebrities. In 1760, founder James Henry Creed established his firm in London. In 1854, the firm moved to Paris and continued to flourish under the tutelage of Creed descendants. Today Olivier Creed, master perfumer and president, carries on the family business.

Jan's Note: One of my fellow writer friends, Allison Pataki, has penned a fascinating historical novel based on the Empress "Sisi" aptly entitled *The Accidental Empress*, which she followed with another book, *Sisi: Empress On Her Own*. Allison wrote about Sisi's dedication to her flowing tresses so it's interesting to imagine her hair perfumed with Fantasia de Fleurs.

Vintage Perfumes

Scent Type: Classic Floral
Top Notes: Bergamot
Heart Notes: Bulgarian rose, Florentine iris
Base Notes: Ambergris infusion

Who's Worn It
Empress Elisabeth of Austria-Hungary "Sisi", Isabelle Adjani

Introduced: 1862

***

Farouche
Nina Ricci

Celebrate the splendor of Paris. Farouche is a feminine floral bouquet from the Paris-based house of Nina Ricci, a firm established in 1932 by the designer and her son, Robert Ricci, who headed the perfume division.

Created in 1974, Farouche has attained classic status in the world of perfumery. In the opening chords, mandarin and galbanum form a spirited green impression. An effusive floral melody follows featuring lily, rose, carnation, honeysuckle, iris, and jasmine. In the finale, soft sandalwood and oakmoss create a lingering aura that whispers of wealth and sensuality.

Inspired by the ever romantic, ever chic City of Light, Farouche is a French-accented fragrance for romantics at heart. The line's exquisite heart-shaped bottles are a Valentine ode to perfumery.

Jan's Note: Farouche is another vintage perfume that is part of Nina Ricci's prestige collection. If you have trouble finding it, look to the company online.

Scent Type: Powdery Floral
Top Notes: Peach, bergamot, green notes, aldehydes
Heart Notes: Rose, carnation, cyclamen, geranium
Base Notes: Musk, sandalwood, vetiver, amber

Introduced: 1974

***

Femme
Rochas

Femme is a full-bodied fragrance from Parfums Rochas, a fragrance as rich in history as in scent. The distinctive composition was created for the House of Rochas during World War II by the noted perfumer Edmond Roudnitska of Cabris, France. When once asked about his olfactory gift, Roudnitska replied, "The capacity to create is essentially the ability to imagine." To the perfumer, the fragrance is a composition as evocative as a Monet masterpiece.

Marcel Rochas opened his couture salon in Paris in 1924 and quickly became known for his broad-shouldered suits, bustiers, and elaborate designs. Femme was originally available only by strict invitation. Rochas sent a letter to his clients allowing them to purchase a limited-edition, numbered bottle. Imagine the demand he created. The next year when he made Femme available to the public, he had an instant hit.

The legendary Femme explodes with Mediterranean fruits, mingled with intoxicating floral aromas, and underscored with lingering balsamics and moss. Femme is a brilliant, recognizable fragrance.

The bottle, designed by René Lalique, is a sensuously curved crystal flacon symbolic of a woman's graceful silhouette. The voluptuous Mae West, who was a personal friend of Lalique and a valued client of Rochas, inspired the bottle. Our favorite Mae West quote is: "Between two evils, I always pick the one I never tried before."

Femme—created to embody femininity.

Jan's Note: Like many vintage perfumes that have been reformulated to meet European Union requirements, Femme has also undergone a reorchestration. The floral heart remains, yet woods seem more prominent. Though altered—and what remains truly unaltered since World War II?—Femme is still immensely enjoyable.

Scent Type: Chypre – Fruity
Top Notes: Peach, plum, bergamot, lemon, rosewood
Heart Notes: Ylang-ylang, jasmine, May rose, clove, orris
Base Notes: Musk, amber, oakmoss, vanilla, patchouli, benzoin, leather

Who's Worn It
Mae West, Audrey Hepburn, Elizabeth Taylor

Introduced: 1944

***

Fidji
Guy Laroche

Fidji was introduced by fashion designer Guy Laroche and created by perfumer Josephine Catapano. The fragrance borrows its name from the Fiji Islands in the South Pacific.

Appropriately, the fragrance opens with fresh tropical notes, evolving into a radiant floral heart. A mild base of fragrant woods produces a soft powdery drydown, reminiscent of tropical island gardens.

Scent Type: Floral
Top Notes: Galbanum, hyacinth, lemon, bergamot
Heart Notes: Carnation, orris, ylang-ylang, jasmine, rose
Base Notes: Vetiver, musk, moss, sandalwood

Vintage Perfumes

Introduced: 1966

***

Fille d'Eve
Nina Ricci

Love in the Garden of Eden. Fille d'Eve is a beloved vintage favorite from the firm established by French couturier Nina Ricci and her son, Robert Ricci. The creative duo achieved brilliance with an earlier fragrance, the classic L'Air du Temps.

Jasmine, sensual and enchanting, blooms in the heart of the magical bouquet. Exotic vetiver and warm oakmoss form a sophisticated finish that regales the senses. The fragrant "love apple" resides in a frosted apple-shaped bottle designed by Marc Lalique.

Scent Type: Chypre
Top Notes: Oakmoss, vetiver
Heart Notes: Jasmine
Base Notes: Oakmoss, vetiver

Introduced: 1952

***

Fiori di Capri
Carthusia

Carnation grows wild on the idyllic island of Capri where, through the magic of alchemy, one of the world's tiniest perfumeries turns handpicked flowers into Fiori di Capri, a rich feminine fragrance redolent of carnation.

From the Italian firm of Carthusia, Fiori di Capri is a romantic elixir that brings to mind carefree Mediterranean holidays. The sensual floral fragrance is blended from Capri's natural island harvest including carnation, which takes center stage, along with ylang-ylang and lily of the valley. Sandalwood and oak serve up smooth refinement—with a side of spirituality.

According to legend, monks of the Carthusian Monastery of St. Giacomo blended the original Capri perfumes in the 14th century. In 1948, the Father Prior discovered the ancient formulas. With the Pope's permission, hand production began using the island's natural flora and vintage methods. Today, the tiny perfumery of Carthusia produces its line in accordance with tradition.

Scent Type: Classic Floral
Top Notes: Lily of the valley
Heart Notes: Carnation, ylang-ylang
Base Notes: Oak, Sandalwood, Amber

Vintage Perfumes

Who's Worn It
Jacqueline Kennedy Onassis

Introduced: 1948

***

First
Van Cleef & Arpels

First-class fragrance. First is an elegant floral bouquet from world-renowned Parisian jeweler Van Cleef & Arpels. A classic fragrance, First was inducted into The Fragrance Foundation's Hall of Fame, an honor awarded to few brands.

Created by perfumer Jean-Claude Ellena, First is elegant and sophisticated. Its sparkling notes create a brilliant, jewel-like aromatic shimmer. A beautiful bouquet of jasmine, rose, and narcissus softens into a powdery amber-sandalwood finish that cloaks the skin like a silken veil with a dark hint of mystery underneath.

First is housed in a lovely curved glass bottle bearing a gold-colored pinafore inscribed with the name and capped with a rounded, easy-to-grasp stopper.

First conjures images of diamonds and platinum, of wealth and privilege. It is a grand floral perfume, a triumph of femininity. When getting dressed for a night on the town, remember: fragrance First, jewels last. Gives a whole new meaning to the concept of layering, *n'est-ce pas?*

JAN MORAN

Jan's Note: Few luxury experiences can compare to entering the luxurious abode of Van Cleef & Arpels in Paris, situated across from the Ritz Hotel in the wide Place Vendôme. I suppose it helped to arrive in a chauffeured car (we were returning from a meeting at Sephora headquarters), but the staff rolled out the red carpet for us. There's something quite heady about trying on million-dollar canary diamonds. Though temporarily out of my budget, I'll certainly settle quite happily for First, an exquisite perfume that shall forever remind me of Paris and the Place Vendôme.

Scent Type: Powdery Floral
Top Notes: Aldehydes, mandarin, black currant bud, peach, raspberry, hyacinth
Heart Notes: Turkish rose, narcissus, jasmine, lily of the valley, carnation, orchid, tuberose, orris
Base Notes: Amber, tonka bean, oakmoss, sandalwood, vetiver, musk, honey, civet

Introduced: 1976

***

Vintage Perfumes

Fleurissimo
Creed

The Paris-based House of Creed has created masterpiece perfumes for royalty, dignitaries and celebrities from around the world, including the courts of England, Spain, and France, since 1760.

In 1972, while awaiting his marriage to American actress Grace Kelly, Prince Rainier of Monaco commissioned from Creed a perfume for his bride to wear on their wedding day. Thus was born Fleurissimo, the perfume created for Her Serene Highness Princess Grace of Monaco.

A fragrance fit for a princess, Fleurissimo is a subtly intoxicating bouquet of delicate white flowers. Feminine and beguiling, versatile and easy to wear, the pedigreed eau de parfum exudes privilege, wealth, and a world of infinite possibilities. Fleurissimo is a majestic scent, once worn exclusively by a legendary woman of international acclaim.

Jan's Note: One spring while visiting Cannes, a friend and I ventured out on an impromptu visit to Monaco. We wound through snaking streets, visited the grand casino, and dined aboard a private yacht in the harbor. Later, we found ourselves en route to the palace. Only then, as I stood before the palace, did it dawn on me—that morning I had unconsciously applied Fleurissimo.

JAN MORAN

Scent Type: Floral
Notes: Tuberose, violet, rose, iris

Who's Worn It
Princess Grace of Monaco, Queen Elizabeth II, Cindy Crawford, Madonna, Rita Wilson, Jacqueline Kennedy Onassis

Introduced: 1972

***

Fleurs de Bulgarie
Creed

The Paris-based house of Creed has long created masterpiece perfumes for royalty, dignitaries, and celebrities. Created by Creed in 1845 for the English Queen Victoria, and reintroduced in 1980, Fleurs de Bulgarie remains a classic.

The rich, romantic Bulgarian rose bouquet is underscored with musk and ambergris. Beguiling and sophisticated, its allure is legendary.

Jan's Note: Bulgaria is one of the largest producers of rose oil in the world. In fact, should you ever find yourself in Bulgaria, visit Rose Valley, also known as the Valley of Roses, where a Festival of Roses is held in Kazanlak every summer. The fields are a fragrant sight to behold.

Vintage Perfumes

Scent Type: Classic Floral
Top Notes: Bergamot
Heart Notes: Bulgarian rose
Base Notes: Ambergris infusion, musk

Who's Worn It
Queen Victoria, Marie Osmond

Introduced: 1845

***

Fleurs de Rocaille
Caron

Fleurs de Rocaille is another timeless scent from the great Parisian perfumery of Caron. It is an enduring floral blend centered on the classic carnation. It was introduced in an upturned glass bottle tied with a gold-colored ribbon beneath a crystal stopper. Sophisticated simplicity in the style of white pearls and twin-sets.

In addition, Fleurs de Rocaille enjoyed a Hollywood walk-on role in the movie *Scent of a Woman*. Al Pacino portrays a rough-hewn military man who has lost his sight and his will to live. At the end of the movie, when he finally decides to choose life, he meets a woman and is enchanted by her as well as her fragrance—Fleurs de Rocaille. With one deep breath he identifies the scent, and to him it represents the captivating scent of a woman.

The power of the movies...in just one scene, an entire new generation became acquainted with the vintage Fleurs de Rocaille.

Jan's Note: In a confusing move, Caron created a newer version called Fleur de Rocaille, which is presumably only one flower, rather than a handful. It's a lighter edition that revolves around lily of the valley, an ethereal scent. Rather different, but carrying such similar names as to cause eternal confusion.

Scent Type: Floral
Top Notes: Lily of the valley, clover
Heart Notes: Rose, violet, lilac, jasmine, iris
Base Notes: Sandalwood, musk, civet

Who's Worn It
Beyoncé Knowles

Introduced: 1933
***

Folavril

Annick Goutal

Annick Goutal's Folavril was one of the first perfumes she created. Folavril bursts with naturally fresh citrus and floral notes, smoothed with tropical mango. In French,

Vintage Perfumes

Folavril loosely translates as "fool's folly."

An accomplished pianist and model, Annick Goutal fell in love with perfumery in the late 1970s and began to blend her own perfumes. She launched her line in the early 1980s and continued to expand her company, which was later acquired. After her early demise in 1999, her daughter, Camille, stepped into her mother's creative role.

Jan's Note: Try blending Annick Goutal fragrances to create your own interpretations. For example, give Folavril a crisp lift by marrying it with Goutal's citrusy chypre Eau d'Hadrien.

Scent Type: Floral - Fruity
Notes: Jasmine, mango, citrus

Who's Worn It
Jeanne Moreau, Sylvie Vartan, Isabelle Huppert, Juliette Greco

Introduced: 1981

***

JAN MORAN

Fracas
Robert Piguet

Fracas, by Parisian couturier Robert Piguet, is a classic French floral bouquet bursting with the white flowers for which Grasse is famous. Fracas, meaning "violent noise" in French, is a brilliant portrait of tuberose, an expansive white floral. The tuberose flower has a scent so intense a single stalk will drench a room with its intoxicating, sensual aroma. Legendary female perfumer Germaine Cellier created Fracas which was launched just after World War II.

Piguet was known for his designs of unerring style and simple elegance. During World War II, Nazi orders directed the top couture houses to relocate to Berlin. Piguet rebelled and resisted and rode out the war in occupied Paris while continuing his work in fashion and fragrance. During this period he commissioned Fracas and Bandit, fragrant points of light in a dark time of history. After a lengthy absence, both fragrances were revived according to their original versions and reintroduced, gaining large celebrity followings.

Swiss by birth, Piguet moved to France at seventeen to pursue his dreams. After working with Redfern and Paul Poiret, he set out on his own. His salon on the prestigious Rond Point des Champs-Élysées catered to an exclusive clientele and was one of the most exclusive destinations for style in Paris. Under his tutelage, other young designers learned their craft and gained their wings, including Hubert

Vintage Perfumes

de Givenchy, Pierre Balmain, and James Galanos.

Heady, mysterious, frank sensuality—the hallmark of Fracas is obvious. Look for Fracas in a black glass cube with simple pink accents. Retro-glamour at its finest.

Jan's Note: Quite simply one of the finest tuberose perfumes in history and the definition of a high quality luxury perfume. Deep appreciation to the fine team who revived the artistry of Robert Piguet and Germaine Cellier perfumes.

Scent Type: Floral
Top Notes: Bergamot, mandarin, hyacinth, greens
Heart Notes: Tuberose, jasmine, orange flower, lily of the valley, white iris, violet, jonquil, carnation, coriander, peach, osmanthus, pink geranium
Base Notes: Musk, sandalwood, orris, vetiver, tolu balsam

Who's Worn It
Princess Caroline of Monaco, Kim Basinger, Edie Sedgwick, Madonna, Courtney Love, Iman, Amanda Harlech, Morgan Fairchild, Kerry Washington, Carolina Herrera, Sophie Dahl Stella Tennant, Debi Mazer, Beverly Sills, Martha Stewart, Sarah Michelle Gellar, Kate Beckinsale, Dita Von Teese, Marlene Dietrich, Sofia Coppola

Introduced: 1948

Gardénia
Chanel

Coco Chanel's twenties version of Gardénia is a polished floral blend enhanced by a spicy accord and supported by sweet, powdery wooded notes. Originally created by perfumer Ernest Beaux, Gardénia is the light, unforgettable essence of springtime gardens.

Perfect for garden tea or a two-Evian power lunch. We imagine Chanel slipped Gardénia in her suitcase for her frequent French Riviera vacations.

Jan's Note: The Chanel modern recreation of Gardénia remains as faithful as possible to Beaux's vintage perfumes given the European Union restrictions on ingredients. Gardénia is hard to find, unless you know where to look for it; the fragrance is usually available only at the Chanel boutiques.

Scent Type: Floral
Top Notes: Absolutes of jasmine, gardenia, orange blossom, tuberose
Heart Notes: Clove, sage, pimiento
Base Notes: Musk, patchouli, sandalwood, vetiver

Introduced: 1925

***

Vintage Perfumes

Gardénia Passion
Annick Goutal

Talented French perfumer Annick Goutal is the genius behind Gardénia Passion. The scent is a heady harmony of gardenia with leafy green notes but also strongly reminiscent of tuberose. An intense, dramatic, unforgettable composition. If you wish to lighten this fragrance for summer heat, spritz a finishing layer of Eau d'Hadrien to add a fresh citrus dimension.

Goutal packaging is pure glamour: A limited-edition Louis XVI Baccarat flacon may be filled with a choice of Gardénia Passion or Eau d'Hadrien. The bottle is hand decorated with delicate gold-colored flowers, topped with an old-fashioned atomizer spray, and beautifully presented in a velvet jewelry box with gold-colored cord accents. Utterly exquisite.

Jan's Note: For those with a passion for gardenia and white floral perfumes, Gardénia Passion is not to be missed. Although it is one of the newer fragrances in this book (a mere babe at 26 years old at the time of publication), I included it because Annick Goutal infused her perfumes with such love and vintage character.

Scent Type: Floral
Notes: Gardenia, leafy green notes

Who's Worn It
Liv Tyler, Oprah Winfrey, Rosanna Arquette, Linda Evangelista, Melanie Griffith

Introduced: 1990

***

Giorgio
Giorgio Beverly Hills

Gale and Fred Hayman found immediate success with Giorgio, named after their internationally famous boutique on Rodeo Drive in the heart of Beverly Hills. The heady, exotic floral fragrance that Gale personally oversaw is a glamorous long-lasting scent, so much so that it was banned at some restaurants which spurred it on to even greater success. One of the best-selling fragrances of all times, Giorgio is dramatic and lavish, saucy and full of sexy verve.

Giorgio set the stage for blockbuster fragrance hits of the 1980s and 1990s. The distinctive line, in its yellow and white striped packages, was unveiled at a million-dollar party. It was originally available only at the Rodeo Drive boutique and through mail order. Now, this bestseller can be found virtually worldwide. It is often copied, but never duplicated.

After years of hard work, entrepreneurs Gale and Fred

Vintage Perfumes

Hayman sold the Giorgio Beverly Hills company for a handsome profit when they divorced. But the fragrance remains true to their vision.

Jan's Note: After writing my first book, *Fabulous Fragrances*, I approached Gale Hayman about writing the forward to the book, a task she graciously accepted. I was delighted because I'd always admired Gale's accomplishments as well as her lovely, unerring sense of style.

Scent Type: Floral
Top Notes: Bergamot, mandarin, galbanum, greens, fruits
Heart Notes: Jasmine, rose, carnation, ylang-ylang, orris, lily of the valley, hyacinth
Base Notes: Sandalwood, cedarwood, musk, moss, amber

Who's Worn It
Nancy Reagan, Jacqueline Bisset, Aly Spencer

Introduced: 1982

***

Givenchy III
Givenchy

Givenchy reintroduced one of its legendary perfumes, Givenchy III, which was one of the first widely distributed Givenchy perfumes. Created under the tutelage of French couturier Hubert de Givenchy and named after the numeral address of the Givenchy salon on the exclusive Avenue George V in Paris, Givenchy III evokes the vintage glamour and refinement of early Givenchy couture creations.

Givenchy's Mythical Fragrance Collection is a reintroduction of several beloved vintage perfumes including Givenchy III, Le De, Extravagance, Indecence, and L'Interdit. The Givenchy III rendition is a lovely woodsy mossy chypre blend. Brilliant green galbanum and hyacinth and a rich leathery patchouli finish form an enigmatic impression that lingers beautifully on the skin. Elegant and sophisticated, Givenchy III is a connoisseur's perfume.

Jan's Note: It's widely known that Audrey Hepburn was a close friend of Hubert de Givenchy and often a muse to his creative genius. But did you know that he designed the chic little black dress she wore in *Breakfast at Tiffany's*? Or that the dress sold at auction for the queenly price of $920,000? The dress remains one of the most expensive pieces of movie memorabilia to date.

Vintage Perfumes

Scent Type: Chypre - Floral
Top Notes: Galbanum, hyacinth
Heart Notes: Oriental rose, jasmine
Base Notes: Oakmoss, patchouli

Introduced: 1970

***

Green Irish Tweed
Creed

Green Irish Tweed was created by perfumer Pierre Bourdan for Creed for the elegant, clever-witted actor Cary Grant which speaks volumes for the fragrance, its attitude, and its character. Casually elegant, fresh and sporty, Green Irish Tweed moves with ease through the vagaries of life. Creed often blended special fragrances for clients, and some were allowed to be sold later as was the case with Green Irish Tweed.

The perfumer weaves the green freshness of violet leaves with the powdery root of iris, sandalwood, and ambergris. Harmonious and genial, Green Irish Tweed develops on the skin as comfortably as a favorite tweed jacket.

Designed for men, but many women wear it, too.

Scent Type: Green
Top Notes: Violet leaves, verbena
Heart Notes: Iris, apple
Base Notes: Sandalwood, ambergris

Who's Worn It
Naomi Campbell, Cary Grant, Prince Charles of Wales, Robert Redford, Richard Gere, Quincy Jones, Clint Eastwood

Introduced: 1985

***

Habanita
Molinard

Habanita is a warm Oriental blend from the Paris House of Molinard. Fruity top notes introduce the composition which proceeds through rich florals to a final balsamic drydown of amber, leather, vanilla, and musk. Sweet and sensual, beautiful for evening and cool crisp days.

The original Molinard was established in Grasse in 1849 to supply wealthy vacationers and royalty, including Queen Victoria. A Paris presence was later established. The Grasse factory is now open for tours at certain times of the year. (60 blvd Victor-Hugo, telephone 93-36-01-62. Call ahead to the tourist office; this is a real treat.)

Jan's Note: Habanita is the crown jewel of Molinard, and a fragrance so beloved I was often asked to bring bottles home from my visits to France. If you adore vanilla-based fragrances, this is a vintage worth trying.

Scent Type: Vanilla-Ambery Oriental
Top Notes: Bergamot, peach, orange blossom, raspberry
Heart Notes: Rose, jasmine, ylang-ylang, orris, heliotrope, lilac
Base Notes: Amber, oakmoss, leather, vanilla, musk, cedarwood, benzoin

Who's Worn It
Debi Mazer

Introduced: 1921

***

Habit Rouge
Guerlain

Guerlain's Habit Rouge, translated from French as "red hunting coat," was inspired by a rider's red habit. Blended by perfumer Jean-Paul Guerlain, the fragrance has attained classic status. An Oriental blend of verve and vitality, Habit Rouge opens with fresh citrus top notes, then meanders along a sweet spicy path of orange flower and opopanax to a base of vanilla and patchouli, finally leaving a leathery, individualistic impression.

A weighty rectangular bottle captures the intoxicating essence. Habit Rouge is a fine selection for gentlemen of taste and refinement who appreciate the sensuality and subtlety of Guerlain formulations. And, quite naturally, it's the ideal fragrance for a rousing morning of horse riding.

In addition, women are often known to "borrow" this delicious warm fragrance.

Scent Type: Spicy-Woody Oriental
Top Notes: Bergamot, orange
Heart Notes: Spices, patchouli, orange flower, opopanax
Base Notes: Vanilla, leather,

Who's Worn It
Robert Redford, Alec Baldwin, Richard Gere

Introduced: 1965
***

Indiscret
Lucien Lelong

Indiscret is one of the great classic fragrances of the twentieth century and the legacy of Lucien Lelong, renowned French couturier. Introduced in 1936, this magnificent perfume faded from the scene after Lelong's death but was lovingly resurrected in 1997 by Lelong perfume and couture collectors Arnold Hayward Neis and his wife, Lucy de Puig Neis.

Rich and dramatic, Indiscret is a fragrance of impeccable pedigree. After being awarded the French *Croix de Guerre* for his efforts in World War I, Lucien Lelong opened his first *maison de couture* in 1919. By 1937, he was elected president of the French Fashion Syndicate, the *Chambre Syndicale de la Couture Française*.

While Nazi troops occupied France from 1940 to 1945, Lelong toiled to keep the French fashion industry alive by foiling German attempts to move the industry to Berlin. He is widely credited with maintaining the fashion industry in Paris during World War II and, in the process, keeping some three hundred thousand people employed. Among Lelong's staff were Hubert de Givenchy, Christian Dior, and Pierre Balmain who later made their own marks in the world of fashion and fragrance.

In 1924, Lelong embarked upon his fragrant journey establishing the *Societé des Parfums Lucien Lelong*. A prolific entrepreneur, he created more than twenty-five fragrances. Among them were lettered scents: N (for his wife, Princess Nathalie Paley), J, L, A, B, and C. Many of his fragrances masqueraded under different names in English-speaking markets: La Première (Opening Night), Orgueil (Pride), Joli Bouquet (Pretty Bouquet), Murmure (Whisper), and Mon Image (My Image). One of the most popular of these scents was Indiscret, the scent Arnold and Lucy Neis chose to commemorate the ideals of Lucien Lelong.

Indiscret was reformulated with care by the French perfume house of Mane. The dramatic soul of the original formula created by master perfumer Jean Carles (and mentor to other greats, including Jacques Polge) prevails. Yesteryear's glamour is artfully blended with a new, modern attitude. The result is sensual, captivating, expressive, and sophisticated.

Indiscret features fresh top notes of mandarin, orange blossom and orange flower, with a green lift of galbanum. Following is an intensely feminine heart of jasmine, rose, and tuberose with a twist of cypress and violet leaves. A sultry finish of sandalwood, amber, and vetiver lingers beautifully on the skin. Indiscret is a fragrance for the art of grand living.

A sculptor and glass collector, Lelong favored glass for his bottle designs. Most of Lelong's many and varied bottles are priceless collectibles today. In designing the Indiscret bottle, Lelong draped a silk handkerchief and said, "That is how I want the Indiscret bottle to look—as if they were folds of classical drapery." Bottle designer Marc Rosen served as a consultant in the re-creation of the Indiscret bottle. Faithful to Lelong's original vision, Indiscret is captured in a frosted glass bottle then nestled in brilliant fuchsia satin and boxed in shades of black and gold.

Jan's Note: With deep admiration, this author bids a fond *adieu* to the man who left this world the day she entered it. Perhaps we passed in the corridor of life.

Vintage Perfumes

Scent Type: Floral – Fruity
Top Notes: Mandarin, bergamot, galbanum, orange flower, tiger orchid, white peach blossom, orange blossom
Heart Notes: Jasmine, tuberose, rose, rose geranium, basil, cypress, ylang-ylang, clove, iris, violet leaves
Base Notes: Sandalwood, amber, oakmoss, vetiver, patchouli, white musk, guaiac wood

Who's Worn It
Princess Nathalie Paley, Marlene Dietrich

Introduced: 1936

***

Infini

Caron

More than a century ago in 1912, Ernest Daltroff, a perfumer and founder of Caron, created Infini—a forever fragrance, in French, for the "infinite."

Infini for women was relaunched in 1970 in tribute to the modern age of space travel. Scintillating aldehydes enhance the rich heart of jasmine, rose, lily, and tuberose. Tonka bean and sandalwood add depth and intrigue to this soft, yet tenacious, floral orchestration. A timeless fragrance, Infini celebrates the modern age with great finesse.

Bottle designer Serge Mansau conceived the current angular bottle. The clear glass flacon has crisp, asymmetrical lines with a diamond-shaped cutout in the heart matched by another diamond cutout in the crystal stopper.

Jan's Note: In 1904, perfumer Ernest Daltroff established the house of Caron, and at one time in Paris the two great perfume houses were Caron and Guerlain. Renowned for his artistry, Daltroff created some the world's most enchanting perfumes for women and men, including Narcisse Noir, Nuit de Noel, and Pour Un Homme. Today, under the guidance of a new owner, the house of Caron continues to produce Daltroff's vintage line along with new Caron creations. Post reorchestration, Infini is a brighter, more modern edition of the vintage fragrance.

Scent Type: Powdery Floral
Top Notes: Aldehydes, peach, bergamot, neroli, coriander
Heart Notes: Rose, jasmine, lily of the valley, carnation, ylang-ylang, orris
Base Notes: Sandalwood, musk, vetiver, civet, tonka bean

Introduced: 1912

***

Ivoire
Balmain

The original Ivoire was a 1979 creation, and today's new edition is an elegant version. Couturier Pierre Balmain was inspired by a woman at a gala who was dressed in creamy pale silk, stark among a sea of black tuxedos. After working with fashion legends Christian Dior, Lucien Lelong, Robert Piguet, and Edward Molyneux, Balmain opened his boutique in Paris in 1946 where his designs were sought after by a privileged clientele. Before his death in 1982, he was honored as an Officer of the Legion of Honor, one of France's most esteemed positions.

The classic green formulation of Ivoire from 1979 was reformulated in 2012. Perfumers Jacques and Michel Almairac recreated this classic fragrance, and in the process gave it a much needed facelift. Kudos to this talented team for maintaining the elegance of Ivoire and bringing it into a new century with a touch of grace.

Jan's Note: The modern chypre (mossy woody) is a lightened blend of fresh green notes and soft florals including orange blossom, ylang-ylang, and jasmine. Ivoire is a refined classic, an Audrey Hepburn in *Breakfast at Tiffany's* sort of fragrance that begs to be taken out on the town.

Scent Type: Chypre
Top Notes: Mandarin, violet leaves, galbanum
Heart Notes: Orange blossom, rose, jasmine, ylang-ylang
Base Notes: Cedarwood, pepper, patchouli, vetiver, vanilla

Introduced: 1979

JAN MORAN

Je Reviens
Worth

The couture house of Worth's Je Reviens has been popular for more than sixty years. The fragrance opens with powdered aldehydic top notes before meandering along a floral path doused with rare spices. Smoky incense and mellow amber linger long after the company has gone home.

Englishman Charles Frederick Worth established his fashion salon in Paris 1858 catering to a clientele of wealth and royalty, including the Empress Eugénie. From his shop on the chic rue de la Paix, he saw clients by personal referral only. Flowing, fluid garments became his trademark. His sons, Jean-Philippe and Gaston Worth, continued the business and created fragrances to give to clients, scents that proved so popular they were soon sold on a wider scale, an endeavor managed by great-grandson Roger Worth.

Je Reviens means "I will return." And it does, again and again. A perennial favorite. Look for Je Reviens in the blue aquamarine boxes.

Scent Type: Powdery Floral
Top Notes: Orange blossom, aldehydes, bergamot, violet
Heart Notes: Clove, rose, jasmine, hyacinth, lilac, orris, ylang-ylang
Base Notes: Amber, incense, tonka bean, vetiver, musk, moss, sandalwood

Vintage Perfumes

Who's Worn It
Jane Asher

Introduced: 1932

***

Jicky
Guerlain

Jicky is a fresh fougère from Guerlain that has endured for more than a century. Citrus, lavender, vanilla, and amber form the dominant accords of the classic fragrance, a scent that is shared by men and women.

The Jicky story began in the 1850s when Aimé Guerlain was living in England studying chemistry and medicine. He fell in love with a woman he nicknamed Jicky. All was bliss until his aging father, Pierre François Pascal, summoned him back to Paris to take over the family business. When he asked for Jicky's hand in marriage, her family would not allow it. He returned to Paris alone and brokenhearted.

More than thirty years later, Aimé Guerlain honored the great love of his life by creating a lavender-vanilla fragrance that bore her nickname. He was proud of the breakthrough modern blend that utilized revolutionary technology in the perfumer's palette.

For the floral notes, he discovered a new solvent technology that produced a potent pure flower essence. For the base accord, he employed another of his discoveries, synthesis, which came from a gum resin called benzoin. From this was extracted vanillin, a substance that shared the dominant theme of natural vanilla but lacked the background complexities. Guerlain found that when he blended vanilla and vanillin for the base note of Jicky, the result was a rounder, full-bodied fragrance. Add a generous amount of citrus, thyme, basil, and rosemary, and the result was Jicky, a new breed of fragrance.

But the year was 1889 and respectable women wore light, single flower scents such as lavender, violet, or rose, or simple bouquets. With its multiple notes of citrus, florals, woods, and spices, Jicky was considered strong and scandalous among proper ladies. The only women who wore such distinctive fragrances were prostitutes who presumably mixed strong fragrances so potential clients could identify them on the dark streets.

Indeed, men appreciated Jicky. Soon men who wanted to be slightly provocative began to wear it. By 1912 women's fashion magazines began to praise it and women embraced the complex fragrance once considered scandalous. Today, more than one hundred years later, the original formula Jicky remains popular with women and men, and Aimé Guerlain's great love is legend.

Jan's Note: More than a century and a quarter later, Jicky remains a masterpiece of perfumery, and the formula is quite close to the original, minus a few European Union restricted ingredients. Still, Jicky is a five-star accomplishment, a fragrance that must be worn at least once in your life to be fully appreciated.

Scent Type: Fougère
Top Notes: Bergamot, lemon, mandarin
Heart Notes: Lavender, thyme, rosemary, basil, orris, tonka bean
Base Notes: Vanilla, amber, benzoin, rosewood, spices, leather

Who's Worn It
Jacqueline Kennedy Onassis, Joan Collins, Brigitte Bardot, Sean Connery, Roger Moore, Kenneth Jay Lane, Sarah Bernhardt

Introduced: 1889

***

Joy
Jean Patou

In 1930, the legendary Joy was introduced as the "costliest perfume in the world." French couturier Jean Patou had set out to create a fragrance "free from all vulgarity" at any cost, as well as "impudent, crazy, and extravagant beyond reason." Indeed, the sumptuous scent created by perfumer Henri Alméras quickly became revered as the world's most extravagant perfume and to this day remains one of the costliest perfumes to produce, according to the Patou firm.

The dominant notes are absolute of jasmine and Bulgarian rose, two of the world's rarest and most expensive essences. Each ounce contains the essence from more than 10,000 jasmine flowers and twenty-eight dozen roses. Lavish quantities of the delicate jasmine and elegant rose are woven into a rich tapestry of more than a hundred essences, resulting in a scent that remains true to Jean Patou's vision. Each vessel of fragrance is still mixed and hand-sealed as it was at its inception in a process that for years was carefully overseen by Jean Kerléo, Patou's internationally recognized in-house perfumer who founded Osmothèque, the scent archive in Versailles. (Kerléo went on to recreate many of the Patou vintage perfumes.)

Jean Patou launched his quest for Joy in 1926 when he took his assistant, cafe society woman Elsa Maxwell, with him to Grasse to work with perfumers on the new scent. Together they searched for a fragrance that would meet the exacting requirements of the best-dressed and most discriminating women of the world, the social leaders and accomplished women of their day. After exhaustive testing they were presented with the formula for Joy, a recipe that called for twice the amount of essential oils that other popular perfumes contained. But alas, the perfumer told them it was too expensive to be commercially viable. That cinched it. Hence was born the "costliest fragrance in the world," and women the world over had to have it.

Joy is timeless; as revered today as it was when it was introduced. It remains a strong, dynamic floral essence with an unmistakable stamp of wealth, breeding, and confidence.

Note: the Joy Eau de Parfum (formerly Eau de Joy) is a different fragrance from the Joy *parfum*. Joy Eau de Parfum is a lighter formulation with a bright burst of aldehydes.

Jan's Note: In a word: Extravagant. Whereas Chanel No. 5 is polished perfection and Shalimar is quietly seductive, Joy is a masterpiece of exuberance, a *joie de vivre* perfume that wants nothing more than to spread the light of happiness.

To my nose, Joy is a lush bouquet of flowers blooming with the brilliance of a springtime garden. It's the aromatic equivalent of a gleeful smile. Extravagant? Sure. But why not live life to the fullest?

Scent Type: Floral
Top Notes: Aldehydes, peach, greens, calyx
Heart Notes: Jasmine, Bulgarian rose, ylang-ylang, orchid, lily of the valley, orris, tuberose
Base Notes: Sandalwood, musk, civet

JAN MORAN

Who's Worn It
Julia Roberts, Vivien Leigh, Marilyn Monroe, Joan Rivers, Mary Pickford, Josephine Baker, Gloria Swanson, Barbara Hutton, Constance Bennett, Elsa Maxwell, Olivia de Haviland, Selma Blair, Wallis Simpson

Introduced: 1930

***

Kiehl's Original Musk
Kiehl's

For years, Kiehl's Original Musk has enchanted legions of fans with its intriguing aroma. Dating from 1920, the oil-based fragrance for women and men was resurrected in the 1950s when it was rediscovered at the company in a container marked "love oil." Actress Kyra Sedgwick is one of its many celebrity fans.

Kiehl's calls Original Musk "our classic signature scent," adding: "Our special Musk 'recipe' begins with an initial creamy, fresh citrus burst of bergamot nectar and orange blossom, followed by a soft bouquet of rose, lily, ylang-ylang, and neroli, a warm, sensual Oriental finish of tonka bean, white patchouli and, of course, musk...the soul of this distinctively modern scent." Revel in the warmth and passion of this timeless unisex fragrance.

Vintage Perfumes

Jan's Note: A favorite underground classic, a simple fragrance with an earthy floral aroma that seduces the senses. A gourmand formula that's almost good enough to eat.

Scent Type: Floral Musk
Top Notes: Orange blossom, bergamot, nectar
Heart Notes: Lily, neroli, rose, ylang-ylang
Base Notes: Musk, patchouli, tonka bean

Who's Worn It
Julianne Moore, Kyra Sedgwick, Natalie Massenet, Rose McGowan, Eugenia Silva, Benjamin McKenzie, Indira Varma

Introduced: 1920

***

L'Air du Temps
Nina Ricci

L'Air du Temps is a classic French fragrance from the Parisian firm of Nina Ricci. The name L'Air du Temps translates as, "the mood of the times, an intangible, like the air we breathe." Ricci's son and business partner, Robert, once said, "For me, perfume is an act of love. A real...or imagined love. I'm a romantic, I can't conceive of life without dreams."

The feminine FiFi Award-winning fragrance is

reminiscent of a bouquet of sun-kissed spring flowers strewn across a bed of precious woods and subtle spices. L'Air du Temps is an easy-to-wear floral scent that floats effortlessly from day to evening. Graceful, feminine, innocent, and understated.

Italian-born Nina Ricci opened her couture boutique in 1932 amidst worldwide uncertainty. Closed in 1939 during World War II, the business reopened six years later under the direction of her son Robert. Before her death in 1970, Nina Ricci was awarded the French Legion of Honor for her collections and accomplishments.

Robert Ricci and Marc Lalique designed the lovely flacon. A pair of doves swoon atop the stopper, wings spread, beaks touching in a timeless image of love. As it was in 1948, the perfume is sold in Lalique flacons of various hues. Perfumer Francis Fabron created the legendary perfume with a lovely lily heart and a warm ambery-sandalwood finish.

Pronounced "lair doo taw," this masterpiece remains a fragrance of infinite romance for lovers the world over. Reorchestrated but still a pleasure to wear.

Scent Type: Floral
Top Notes: Bergamot, peach, rosewood, neroli
Heart Notes: Gardenia, carnation, jasmine, May rose, ylang-ylang, orchid, lily, clove, orris
Base Notes: Ambergris, musk, vetiver, benzoin, cedarwood, moss, sandalwood, spices

Vintage Perfumes

Who's Worn It
Padma Lakshmi, Queen Sophia, Lana Turner, Princess Michael of Kent, Christiane Celle

Introduced: 1948

***

L'Heure Attendue
Jean Patou

In perfumery, French couturier Jean Patou is perhaps most remembered for his incomparable perfumes Joy and 1000. Patou had L'Heure Attendue crafted to celebrate the liberation of Paris from the Nazi occupation during World War II. Formulated to reflect the ensuing *joie de vivre*, it is a spicy Oriental composition with an expansive, freewheeling personality.

At the heart of the perfume is a liberal floral bouquet of jasmine, rose, and ylang-ylang. A spicy finale is warmed with sandalwood, vanilla, and patchouli. The effect is one of joyful exuberance. L'Heure Attendue is a beautiful scent for evening and winter wear, a jubilant scent with the classic verve of yesteryear.

Jan's Note: In 1984, in-house perfumer Jean Kerléo painstakingly recreated the once discontinued L'Heure Attendue, along with other vintage Patou perfumes, adhering strictly to the original formula as much as possible.

Scent Type: Oriental – Spicy
Top Notes: Lily of the valley, geranium, lilac
Heart Notes: Ylang-ylang, jasmine, rose, opopanax
Base Notes: Mysore sandalwood, vanilla, patchouli

Introduced: 1946

***

L'Heure Bleue
Guerlain

L'Heure Bleue means "blue hour" in French, and it was reportedly inspired by the gentle blue-hued twilight of a pre-World War I Paris, a time of relative innocence and appreciation of beauty known as the Belle Époque period which ended with war in 1914.

Third-generation perfumer Jacques Guerlain conceived L'Heure Bleue for the sophisticated woman of 1912. He freely employed the latest synthetic ingredients to create a totally new scent combined with passionate florals of carnation, violet, and orange blossom and dusky base notes of vanilla, musk, and aromatic woods. The resulting gourmand scent is tender yet penetrating, like a twilit evening in Paris with undercurrents of bewitching sensuality and a powdery *sillage*.

The perfume is captured in a heavy glass flacon adorned by scrollwork on the shoulders. The triangular stopper is shaped like a gentleman's hat, a *chapeau de gendarme,* from which a hand-tied silken tassel dangles.

L'Heure Bleue was a landmark scent of 1912 and remains an enchanting favorite. A classic French perfume, L'Heure Bleue is an elegant selection for the romantic at heart.

Jan's Note: L'Heure Bleue is a smooth, velvety perfume that whispers of romance and nostalgia. One of the finest Guerlain perfumes, L'Heure Bleue remains a vintage perfume of masterpiece proportion.

Scent Type: Floral Oriental
Top Notes: Orange blossom, bergamot, aniseed
Heart Notes: Tuberose, violet, Bulgarian rose, carnation
Base Notes: Musk, orange blossom, benzoin, tonka bean, vanilla, iris (orris)

Who's Worn It
Julia Roberts, Kate Moss, Patricia Arquette, Queen Elizabeth II, Carolyn Roehm, Catherine Deneuve, Teri Garr, Liza Minnelli, Bianca Jagger, Jade Jagger, Wendy Wasserstein, Ursula Andress, Pat Nixon

Introduced: 1912
***

L'Interdit
Givenchy

Renowned French couturier Hubert de Givenchy and perfumer Francis Fabron created this aldehydic floral bouquet for actress Audrey Hepburn who became a friend of the designer. It is said that for many years, Hepburn was the only woman allowed to wear the fragrance. Givenchy was one of her favorite designers and created many of her clothes for films such as *Breakfast at Tiffany's*.

L'Interdit is a smooth blend of elegant floral notes in perfect harmony with bright aldehydes and succulent fruits. Balsamic base notes create an understated sensual aura. If fragrance were a movie scene, L'Interdit would be the opening sequence of *Breakfast at Tiffany's* with Hepburn draped in a black Givenchy evening dress gazing into the Tiffany window of sparkling jewels. Quietly alluring, L'Interdit is a fragrance of tasteful sophistication.

In 2007, Givenchy reorchestrated the 1957 floral fragrance (which had also been reformulated prior to 2007). This version of L'Interdit is a return to the vintage original, or as close as it can be today. A powdery soft floral bouquet; the rose heart is freshened with the addition of pink pepper and jasmine. Velvety orris, or iris root, and tonka bean form a suede-soft finish. Very simply, L'Interdit is timeless elegance.

Vintage Perfumes

Jan's Note: L'Interdit is as lovely as the woman for whom it was created. The return to the original formula is welcome, indeed.

Scent Type: Powdery Floral
Top Notes: Aldehydes, bergamot, peach
Heart Notes: Bulgarian rose, jasmine, pink pepper
Base Notes: Iris, tonka bean

Who's Worn It
Audrey Hepburn

Introduced: 1957

***

Lauren
Ralph Lauren

From American designer Ralph Lauren hails a light contemporary, feminine floral fragrance with a snappy apple accent. Lauren opens with energizing greens and fruits followed by a floral harmony of lily of the valley with undertones of spices and woods. Created to augment easy-to-wear Ralph Lauren designs and timeless American classics.

Ralph Lauren explains: "My philosophy about fragrance, like fashion, is simple: Never accept substitutes for the best. And if the best doesn't exist, create it."

The understated fragrance is presented in ruby red

flacons, accented with gold-colored caps. The clear lead crystal perfume flacon was inspired by antique regency inkwells and is now part of the permanent collection of the Cooper-Hewitt Museum in New York.

Scent Type: Floral – Fruity
Top Notes: Wild marigold, apple, greens, rosewood, pineapple
Heart Notes: Bulgarian rose, lilac, violet, jasmine, lily of the valley, cyclamen
Base Notes: Cedarwood, oakmoss, sandalwood, vetiver, carnation

Who's Worn It
Christina Applegate

Introduced: 1978

***

Lavanda Imperiale
Santa Maria Novella

From 1937, Lavanda Imperiale from Italy's Santa Maria Novella is a fresh herbaceous lavender scent with zesty citrus accents.

If you crave the classics, consider the lineage of this fragrance house. Eight hundred years ago an order of Dominican monks established the firm of Santa Maria

Vintage Perfumes

Novella. Today, in a converted neo-Gothic chapel in the heart of Florence, exotic essences continue to entice the senses.

There, perfumers blend pure natural ingredients for creations such as Lavanda Imperiale, a unisex cologne that is the essence of clean.

Scent Type: Fougère Citrus

Notes: Lavender, citrus

Introduced: 1937

***

Le Dix
Balenciaga

Le Dix is a classic fragrance created by perfumer Francis Fabron for the celebrated Spanish couturier Cristobal Balenciaga. The vintage perfume is a creamy blend of violet and powdery aldehydes enriched with a luscious woody theme.

Le Dix debuted in Paris in 1947—the same year Christian Dior introduced his New Look collection of post-World War II fashion. Le Dix was one of the new postwar fragrances eagerly sought out by those who had denied themselves of luxuries for far too long during the war.

Balenciaga was born in northern Spain but moved to

Paris in 1937 during the Spanish Civil War. Creator of the pillbox hat, three-quarter sleeves, and flamenco dresses, he also trained other young designers such as Ungaro and Courrèges. He designed for women of wealth and title, including those of the Spanish royal family. Today, his couture designs reside in the New York Metropolitan Museum collection.

Jan's Note: Le Dix is French for "ten," and the perfume was named for Balenciaga's salon at No. 10, avenue Georges V. It still scores a perfect ten on my vintage list.

Scent Type: Powdery Floral
Top Notes: Aldehydes, peach, lemon, bergamot, coriander
Heart Notes: Jasmine, rose, orris, lilac, lily of the valley
Base Notes: Vetiver, sandalwood, musk, amber, tonka bean, benzoin, Peru balsam

Introduced: 1947

***

Vintage Perfumes

Liù

Guerlain

Every Guerlain fragrance begins with a story, before even the first drop of essential oil is selected. A character from Puccini's opera *Turandot* inspired the delicate Liù.
Liù is a charming romantic fragrance featuring a bouquet of jasmine, rose, and iris, with jasmine as the lead. Fresh citrus and a powdery finish complete the floral aldehyde formula blended by Jacques Guerlain. Inspired by a woman of tenderness and passion, whose love and generosity are boundless, Liù is intentionally understated, a refined, subtle perfume

Guerlain submitted this story of *Turandot*:

In the opera, the Princess Turandot dares any prince or nobleman who seeks her hand in marriage to successfully answer three riddles or be sentenced to death.

One of her suitors, the Unknown Prince, accepts the challenge and proffers triumphant responses to the riddles, thereby winning the Princess's hand. Sensitive to the Princess's opposition to the marriage, however, the Prince offers Turandot a challenge of his own: If she can guess his name, he will relinquish his right to her hand.

The desperate princess kidnaps Timur, the Prince's father, and threatens to torture him until he reveals the guarded secret. To save Timur's life, Liù, the Prince's servant, acknowledges that she is the only one who knows the Prince's name. After admitting to Turandot that she is deeply in love with the Prince, Liù takes her own life, guarding the secret forever.

The Prince grants Turandot one more chance at freedom by divulging his name: Calaf. Moved by Liù's amorous gesture, Turandot proclaims the Prince's true name to be Love.

Scent Type: Powdery Floral
Top Notes: Bergamot, neroli, aldehydes
Heart Notes: Jasmine, May rose, iris
Base Notes: Amber, vanilla, woods

Who's Worn It
Diana Ross, Ethel Kennedy, Rose Kennedy

Introduced: 1929

***

Ma Griffe
Carven

In French, *ma griffe* refers to a signature or personal stamp. Thus, couture designer Carven selected the name for her personal fragrance which was created by perfumer Jean Carles. Ma Griffe is a blend of earthy green essences, a jasmine and rose heart, and the chypre finish of oakmoss and sandalwood. Ma Griffe is a timeless, easy-to-wear classic, steeped in mosses, flowers, and woody balsamics.

Carven made quite a splash with Ma Griffe. When she launched the fragrance, she hired a plane to drop thousands of tiny, parachuted perfume samples across Paris. The response was overwhelming.

Carven founded the House of Carven in 1944. From her Paris salon at the Rond Point des Champs-Élysées, she led the way in creating haute couture especially for petite women; she herself was just five feet tall. Along with her signature samba dresses, silk scarves, furs, and jewelry collections, she sold her fragrance creations. Though Ma Griffe was her personal scent, she also introduced other classics: Robe d'un Soir, Madame Carven, Vert et Blanc, and Variations.

Jan's Note: When my first book on perfume, *Fabulous Fragrances*, was published in 1994, one of the highlights was inscribing a book to Madame Carven, a couture designer I have long admired. Born Carmen de Tommaso and known as Marie-Louise Carven, or simply, Madame Carven, she blazed a successful trail in the post-WWII, male-dominated fashion landscape of Paris, 1945. Her branded name was derived from her first name, Carmen, and her aunt's surname of Boyriven.

Madame Carven lived until the age of 105, departing this world in 2015. Besides her iconic line, she also designed uniforms for twenty airlines and patented the push-up bra.

Here's to an accomplished woman and her life well-lived.

Scent Type: Chypre – Floral
Top Notes: Gardenia, greens, galbanum, aldehydes, clary sage
Heart Notes: Jasmine, rose, sandalwood, vetiver, orris, ylang-ylang
Base Notes: Styrax, oakmoss, cinnamon, musk, benzoin, labdanum

Who's Worn It
Barbara Walters, Leslie Caron, Edith Piaf

Introduced: 1946

***

Magie Noire
Lancôme

From Lancôme comes Magie Noire, or "black magic" in French. Created by perfumer Gerard Goupy, the spicy Oriental blend is as smooth as Far Eastern silk.

Fiery incense and sensual amber warm a classic bouquet of rose and jasmine. For women who love the romance of exotic fragrances, this elixir is sure to enchant. Imagine candlelit dinners and snowy evenings—that's Magie Noire. Bewitching and seductive, it's perfect for conjuring a little night magic.

The round bottle, designed by master bottle designer Pierre Dinand, sports a deeply indented V-shape draped around the shoulders like a plunging neckline.

Scent Type: Spicy Woody Oriental
Top Notes: Hyacinth, cassie, bergamot, raspberry, galbanum
Heart Notes: Jasmine, ylang-ylang, Bulgarian rose, lily of the valley, narcissus, honey, tuberose, orris
Base Notes: Spices, sandalwood, amber, cedarwood, patchouli, oakmoss, musk, civet

Who's Worn It
Isabella Rossellini

Introduced: 1981

***

Mediterraneo Carthusia
Carthusia

On the sunny Mediterranean isle of Capri, one the world's tiniest perfumeries, Carthusia, produces scents blended from island harvests. Dynamic and refreshing, Mediterraneo is a classic citrus formula for women and men.

In Mediterraneo, orchard-fresh lemon leaves and soothing green tea combine with a subtle floral bouquet.

Cedarwood and vetiver form a hearty finish. The veritable soul of Capri, it's an engaging, restorative scent and even comes complete with a papal blessing.

Legend has it that at the Carthusian Monastery of St. Giacomo, 14th century monks blended the original Capri perfumes. In 1948, the Father Prior discovered the ancient formulas. With the Pope's permission, hand production began using the island's natural flora and vintage methods. Once available only on Capri, Mediterraneo is a rare find.

Scent Type: Citrus
Top Notes: Lemon, leaves
Heart Notes: Tea
Base Notes: Vetiver, cedarwood

Who's Worn It
George Clooney

Introduced: 1948

***

Miss Dior
Dior

A classic, impeccable chypre floral fragrance, Miss Dior was created by perfumer Jean Carles for French couturier Christian Dior. The freshness of green galbanum, the exuberance of a floral bouquet, and the leathery oakmoss-

Vintage Perfumes

patchouli finale made Miss Dior a sensation. The fragrance was reportedly named after Dior's younger sister, a fresh-faced ingénue, and conceived to reflect his couture fashion line of the season.

Miss Dior was launched in 1947, the year Dior, a former assistant to couturier Pierre Balmain, introduced his new post-war collection. *Harper's Bazaar* editor-in-chief Carmel Snow called it "The New Look." The style was actually a throwback to the pre-World War II years with full skirts, tiny waistlines, gloves, and bare shoulders. This was a far cry from the despondent styles of the war years. When consumers flocked to update their wardrobes with the New Look, they also snapped up Dior's new fragrance, Miss Dior. The fragrance represented the re-emergence of the feminine, elegant styles of the Belle Époque that many women were eager to return to.

Today, the perennial French debutante Miss Dior is enjoying a resurgence. She bows in a hound's tooth-embossed clear crystal flacon with a pristine white satin bow at her neckline. Miss Dior is still lovely after all these years.

Jan's Note: I have a vintage Miss Dior set that still fills the room with exquisite, graceful complexities. Miss Dior has undergone a number of reorchestrations due to the evolution of ingredient ordinances. The current edition brings forth brisk aldehydic notes in true vintage fashion.

Scent Type: Chypre - Floral
Top Notes: Bergamot, aldehydes, clary sage, gardenia, galbanum
Heart Notes: Rose, jasmine, lily of the valley, carnation, orris
Base Notes: Patchouli, oakmoss, amber, vetiver, sandalwood, leather

Who's Worn It
Princess Margaret of England

Introduced: 1947

***

Mitsouko
Guerlain

Third generation perfumer Jacques Guerlain conceived Mitsouko for women of passion, intensity, strength, and introspection. Created on the eve of the Roaring Twenties, Mitsouko reflects the Far Eastern style that became the rage in the flamboyant years after World War I.

Mitsouko opens with fruity top notes of tangy bergamot and smooth, mellow peach. A lilac blend follows, dissolving into a woody chypre drydown, redolent of vetiver, oakmoss, and amber. Mitsouko is a sensual, voluptuous fragrance, like a dark, full-bodied Cabernet Sauvignon.

Mitsouko means "mystery" in Japanese and was inspired

Vintage Perfumes

by a character in the Claude Farrère novel, *La Bataille*, or *The Battle*. The story revolved around the ill-fated love of an English officer and the wife of the ship's commander, a beautiful Japanese woman named Mitsouko. Farrère had mentioned another Guerlain fragrance, Jicky, in one of his novels, so Jacques Guerlain reciprocated the honor by naming his fragrance after a Farrère character. And so Mitsouko lives on in literature and in perfume. It remains one of the great jewels of the House of Guerlain.

Jan's Note: Very simply, Mitsouko is an enigma. The vintage formula, which I researched and referenced in my historical novel, *Scent of Triumph,* is spare and elegant. Hauntingly sensual, Mitsouko is a balanced, refined chypre, a remarkable masterpiece of timeless artistic achievement. Fortunately, gifted perfumer Eduoard Fléchier reorchestrated Mitsouko to come into compliance with European Union guidelines, and the result is a near perfect replication.

When pressed to name my favorite perfume, Mitsouko is often my reply. (But how can I possibly choose just one?) To me, Mitsouko is silk and cashmere on a moonlit evening with the ripe aroma of peaches wafting on a sultry midnight breeze.

Scent Type: Chypre – Fruity
Top Notes: Peach, bergamot, hesperides
Heart Notes: Lilac, rose, jasmine, ylang-ylang
Base Notes: Vetiver, amber, oakmoss, cinnamon, spices

Who's Worn It
Jade Jagger, Jean Harlow, Ingrid Bergman, Diaghilev, Kiri Te Kanawa, Rosamund Pike

Introduced: 1919

***

Mouchoir de Monsieur
Guerlain

In 1904, French perfumer Jacques Guerlain created a masterpiece in men's perfumery destined for the annals of history. Mouchoir de Monsieur is a distinguished fragrance portrait. Today, the century-old classic remains the gold standard of refined perfumery for men.

The name refers to a gentleman's handkerchief, which was customarily offered to his lady. Men of good breeding scented their handkerchiefs with a discreet scent—thus was born the subtle Mouchoir de Monsieur.

Fresh lavender and bergamot form a zesty opening for the rose-jasmine heart. A dusting of cinnamon spices a silky amber finish enriched with earthy patchouli and sweet vanilla. The result is a warm spicy-woody blend that fully engages the senses.

Mouchoir de Monsieur is an elegant reminder of yesteryear, a fragrance that, like a fine cognac, is enhanced by the passage of time.

Scent Type: Spicy-Woody Oriental
Top Notes: Bergamot, lavender
Heart Notes: Jasmine, rose
Base Notes: Vanilla, amber, patchouli, tonka bean

Who's Worn It
Charlie Chaplin

Introduced: 1904

***

Mûre et Musc
L'Artisan Parfumeur

Mûre et Musc (Blackberry and Musk) is one of L'Artisan Parfumeur's most iconic perfumes. Created by founder and perfumer Jean-François Laporte, Mûre et Musc is a fresh blend of blackberry and musk. The warm fruity aroma is sweetly engaging.

"The success of Mûre et Musc was due to the witty and daring contrast in the structure between sparkling top notes and an enveloping warm evolution of the scent's seductive development on the skin. The first of its kind on the market, it remains a global bestseller and set the benchmark for L'Artisan Parfumeur creativity." – L'Artisan Parfumeur

Jan's Note: Creating and guiding a perfume company and its growth is an effort that requires a talented cast. L'Artisan Parfumeur grew from a fledgling company to an international fashion-lovers' favorite under the expert stewardship of François Duquesne, a legend in the perfume industry who I'm fortunate to call a good friend. Along with his wife Celeste, a celebrity makeup artist, François remains dedicated to the industries of perfume and beauty—and we are all the richer for it.

Scent Type: Citrus & Fruits
Top Notes: Lemon, orange, basil
Heart Notes: Jasmine, blackberry, red berries
Base Notes: Musk, oakmoss

Who's Worn It
Toni Braxton, Jenna Elfman, Ashley Olsen, Sarah Wynter

Introduced: 1978

***

Vintage Perfumes

My Sin
Lanvin

From 1925, My Sin was blended by a Russian perfumer known as Madame Zed for French couturier Jeanne Lanvin. It was an immensely popular fragrance of the Roaring Twenties and continued for several decades before being discontinued in 1988. Little is known about the mysterious Madame Zed who created fourteen perfumes for Mme Lanvin. My Sin and Arpège, were Lanvin's most popular perfumes.

My Sin is a voluptuous perfume centered on a dark, passionate bouquet of jasmine and rose with a powdery finish courtesy of balsam, sandalwood, and vanilla. To truly understand My Sin, put it in perspective of the 1920s. It was a time of loosening social mores, flapper girls, and luxurious fashion.

My Sin is a mysterious woman in a slinky black, bias-cut gown rippling around her legs, a chinchilla thrown over one shoulder, red lips and a gold cigarette holder. Perhaps not politically correct by today's standards, but a dangerous, forbidden, languorous glamour of the Roaring Twenties.

Jan's Note: People who once wore this grand perfume mourned its discontinuation. Today, My Sin, also known as Mon Péché, has been resurrected by Long Lost Perfumes and can be found online. Though the new version has a slightly brighter top note than the original, the drydown is virtually identical.

Scent Type: Powdery Floral
Top Notes: Heliotrope, lemon, neroli, bergamot, aldehydes, carnation, clary sage
Heart Notes: Jasmine, lily of the valley, rose, violet, ylang-ylang, iris (orris), clove
Base Notes: Musk, sandalwood, vanilla, vetiver, tolu balsam, styrax, cedarwood

Who's Worn It
Jayne Mansfield

Introduced: 1925

***

N'Aimez Que Moi
Caron

Vintage allure: Under the banner of Caron, perfumer Ernest Daltroff plied this romantic montage like a lover's gift of candy and flowers. In 1917, N'Aimez Que Moi proved wildly popular with troops and their girlfriends as sweethearts pledged their love before parting. N'Aimez Que Moi translates as "love only me."

The floral fragrance blooms with violet, rose, and lilac. Amber and vanilla create a candied confection sweet as a kiss, tinged with earthy greens.

Having catered to a century of lovers, N'Aimez Que Moi remains a fragrant Valentine for the romantic woman.

Scent Type: Classic Floral
Top Notes: Lilac
Heart Notes: Rose, Violet
Base Notes: Vanilla, oakmoss, musk, amber

Introduced: 1917

***

Nahéma
Guerlain

What becomes a legend? Nahéma, a legendary rose perfume blended by Jean-Paul Guerlain for the French actress, Catherine Deneuve. The Guerlain fragrance unfolds with the smooth freshness of fruit followed by one of the richest rose bouquets in perfumery. Nahéma cradles the beloved rose in a warm balsam-vanilla embrace.

As with most Guerlain fragrances, Nahéma began with a story. A character in Scheherazade's *Thousand and One Nights* inspired the name. There were twin sisters, disparate in nature. Nahéma means "daughter of fire," bold and untamed. Passion and intensity governed one sister while the other was tender and gentle. This duality of nature in the twins served as inspiration for Guerlain's fragrance, a scent that is powerful yet delicate, sensual yet innocent. It's a fragrance for making grand entrances.

Nahéma is presented in a graceful, curvaceous bottle, a circular interplay of elegant simplicity.

Jan's Note: Perfumery experts generally agree that Nahéma is one of most intoxicating perfumes in the oeuvre of Guerlain, as well as among the finest rose-centric perfumes of all time. If you love rose perfumes, Nahéma should be one at the top of your list.

Scent Type: Powdery Floral/Rose
Top Notes: Peach, bergamot, greens, aldehydes
Heart Notes: Rose hyacinth, Bulgarian rose, ylang-ylang, jasmine, lilac, lily of the valley
Base Notes: Passion fruit, Peru balsam, benzoin, vanilla, vetiver, sandalwood

Who's Worn It
Natalie Cole, Madonna, Sigourney Weaver, Joan Jett, Catherine Deneuve

Introduced: 1979
***

Vintage Perfumes

Narcisse Noir
Caron

Created by the great perfumer Ernest Daltroff, founder of Caron, Narcisse Noir is based on the black narcissus, an exotic spring-blooming flower found in China and Persia. An Oriental blend of aromatic woods lends a sensual, lingering aura to the assertive floral arrangement.

In this Art Deco period perfume, a dark blend of jasmine and orange blossom is tinged with the sweet smokiness of sandalwood, and the result is thoroughly engaging. Creamy aromatic woods lend a sensual aura to the rich orange-infused floral arrangement of jasmine, rose, and orange blossom. The result is enigmatic and alluring, a lively cross between tart and sweet.

Narcisse Noir was one of the most important fragrances of 1911, an industrious year in the history of perfumery. Today, it remains a sophisticated classic, a hallmark of modern perfumery. Savor the rich Narcisse Noir for glamorous days and romantic evenings…and get ready for your close-up.

Jan's Note: Perfumer Victoria Frolova shares a little Hollywood history on her blog, Bois de Jasmin, writing that, "The [1950] movie *Sunset Boulevard* enshrined this perfume, when Gloria Swanson pronounced the name in a deep sultry voice, 'Black Narcissus, Narcisse Noir.'"

Scent Type: Floral – Oriental
Top Notes: Orange blossom, bergamot, petitgrain, lemon
Heart Notes: Rose, jasmine, jonquil
Base Notes: Persian black narcissus, musk, civet, sandalwood

Who's Worn It
Madonna, Gloria Swanson

Introduced: 1912

***

Normandie
Jean Patou

The year was 1935, and a swank new ocean liner called the Normandie carried the elite of business and society on its maiden voyage from Le Havre to New York.

A new Atlantic crossing speed record was set, and each first-class passenger received Jean Patou's latest fragrance named in honor of the luxury liner. Patou described the fragrance as warm and determined and packaged it in a miniature flacon surrounded by a replica of the ship. Passengers adored the spicy Oriental scent woven of jasmine, rose, and vanilla.

In perfumery, French couturier Jean Patou is perhaps most remembered for his incomparable perfumes, Joy and 1000. Although Patou is no longer with us, the firm that

Vintage Perfumes

bears his name continues to introduce fine fragrances and revive vintage perfumes.

At the helm of the business Patou's great-nephews Guy and Jean de Moüy continue the family legacy having re-created classic Patou perfumes. Jean de Moüy explains their impetus: "Our greatest desire was for these perfumes to be appreciated by the contemporary counterparts of those women who used to love wearing them; in other words, the most elegant, distinguished and also, more often than not, the most famous women in the world."

With Jean Kerléo, who was the in-house perfumer, they re-created classic fragrances from formulas preserved by their great-uncle, the debonair Jean Patou. Jean de Moüy explains these classics "will give lovers of all things beautiful the opportunity of inhaling the scents of a glamorous and exciting era, famous for its seductive elegance...an era in which Jean Patou became a legend in his own lifetime."

In the 1930s, Patou provided a burl and glass cocktail bar in his salon to amuse the gentlemen while the women were being fitted. Along with the usual libations, an assortment of essential oils was also available to patrons so that they could create their own fragrances. The array of classic Patou fragrances takes us back to this ingenious cocktail bar tradition, reminding us of the excesses of the twenties, of the flamboyant jazz age, of aristocratic summers at the Riviera and Deauville, and of the racy Hispano Suiza automobile Patou motored throughout Europe.

Jan's Note: While researching ships from the first half of the 20th century for my historical novel, *Scent of Triumph*, imagine my delight when I discovered a woman who had an original bottle of Normandie from the ship's maiden voyage. It was kismet, no doubt.

Scent Type: Oriental – Ambery
Top Notes: Fruits
Heart Notes: Carnation, jasmine, rose
Base Notes: Vanilla, benzoin, oakmoss, cedarwood, woods

Introduced: 1935

***

Nuit de Noël
Caron

An exotic Oriental fragrance from the House of Caron, Nuit de Noël, which refers to Christmas night or Christmas Eve, begins with exhilarating citrus top notes, followed by a heart of rare flowers. Orris adds a subtle violet-like note to the composition, while sweet vanilla, earthy oakmoss, and balsamic sandalwood form a creamy lasting aura. Nuit de Noël is a fitting fragrance for glittery holiday galas, or a romantic Christmas Eve relaxing with a loved one by a crackling fireplace.

Created in 1922, this classic is presented in a splendid black flacon, designed to accentuate the image of the

Vintage Perfumes

dramatic scent. Close your eyes and inhale and relive a cherished perfume of the Roaring Twenties.

Jan's Note: One of my most treasured vintage perfume finds is a small black bottle of Nuit de Noel ensconced in a sleekly molded, tasseled box covered with jade green and gold print paper, just slim enough to fit into an evening purse. And the aroma? Still rich and divine…nearly a century later.

Scent Type: Oriental
Top Notes: Citrus
Heart Notes: Rose, orris, jasmine, ylang-ylang
Base Notes: Sandalwood, vanilla, oakmoss

Who's Worn It
Andrea Marcovicci

Introduced: 1922

***

Old Spice
Procter & Gamble

Since 1937, Old Spice has graced many a man's dressing table. Originated by the founder of Shulton, William Lightfoot Shultz, the scent is a beloved classic. The spicy fougère blend combines classic elements of citrus, lavender, and oakmoss. Delicious culinary spices set it apart in the fougère category. Nutmeg, vanilla, and incense are supported by velvety amber while sandalwood, patchouli, and vetiver provide an earthy wooded base that launches memories of exotic ports of call.

Old Spice has reinvigorated the brand to appeal to younger men (because once upon a time everyone's grandfather wore it), but the fact is that Old Spice is a surprisingly good fragrance—and you have to love the price. Even women have been known to nab this one.

A mass-market fragrance, Old Spice is well-priced and simply packaged in a creamy porcelain-style bottle with a sketch of a tall-masted sailing ship.

Wear Old Spice in memory of the good old days, or the hunky Old Spice guy on television commercials.

Jan's Note: The sketches of tall-masted ships on Old Spice bottles were drawn from real ships. Here's what a Wikipedia entry has to say: "The original ships used on the packaging were the Grand Turk and the Friendship. Other ships used on Old Spice packaging include the John Wesley, Salem, Birmingham, Maria Teresa, Propontis, Recovery, Sooloo, Star of the West, Constitution, Java, United States, and Hamilton."

Vintage Perfumes

Scent Type: Fougère – Spicy
Top Notes: Bergamot, lemon, carnation, anise, orange
Heart Notes: Lavender, ylang-ylang, cinnamon, jasmine
Base Notes: Amber, incense, vanilla, nutmeg, musk, patchouli, sandalwood, oakmoss, vetiver, tonka bean

Who's Worn It
Bradley Cooper

Introduced: 1937

***

Ombre Rose
Brousseau

Ombre Rose is from Jean-Charles Brousseau, a Parisian couturier known for his expertise in millinery and accessories. Created by perfumer Françoise Caron, the rose floral bouquet is brightened with aldehydes, peach, and geranium then warmed to a powdery finish by sweet vanilla, honey, and exotic woods. Vivid and long-lasting, Ombre Rose is an intense daytime or evening fragrance.

The perfume is housed in a burnished black hexagonal flacon highlighted by a sculpted floral pattern. Other strengths are available in similar bottles of clear glass in bas relief. The bottle designs are based on an antique bottle from Brousseau's personal collection.

Scent Type: Powdery Floral-Rose
Top Notes: Aldehydes, peach, rosewood, geranium
Heart Notes: Lily of the valley, ylang-ylang, rose, orris, sandalwood, cedarwood, vetiver
Base Notes: Vanilla, honey, iris, musk, cinnamon, tonka bean, heliotrope

Introduced: 1981

***

Opium
Yves Saint Laurent

Smoldering and dramatic, Opium is an opulent Oriental blend from French designer Yves Saint Laurent who imagined a perfume for an Asian empress. Created by perfumer Jean-Louis Sieuzac, the fragrance unfolds around a mandarin-accented bouquet of jasmine. Underscoring the composition is an exotic mélange of sweet aromatic woods and incense. Opium is a distinctive fragrance made for grand entrances and seductive evenings.

Opium was a groundbreaking perfume, and so well executed that it won FiFi awards around the world and was inducted into the FiFi Hall of Fame.

Opium caused quite a stir with its controversial name, but the exposure helped to make it a best-selling scent. For the extravagant launch party in 1977, a tall ship, the *Peking*, was rented from the South Street Seaport Museum in New

Vintage Perfumes

York's East Harbor with none other than Truman Capote at the helm. The ship was draped with banners of red, gold, and purple, and the Oriental theme was carried out with a thousand-pound bronze Buddha laden with mounds of white cattleya orchids.

Yves Saint Laurent carried the Oriental theme into the packaging design. The perfume is held in a glass vial encased in a red plastic container inspired by Japanese *inros*. These small lacquered cases were once worn under kimonos on silken cords and held aromatics, herbs, perfumes, and medicines.

"Opium: A window onto an imaginary world. Once upon a time there was Opium - more than just a fragrance, it's an opulent, fascinating, inimitable impression. A one-way ticket to a symbolic and enigmatic faraway place. A dream-like journey into a land of make-believe with unsuspected charm. Experience life at the highest level." —Yves Saint Laurent

Jan's Note: I distinctly recall the moment when I first experienced Opium. A friend had just returned from Martinique and brought the perfume as a gift. It wasn't yet available in the United States, so I latched onto this treasure as if it were gold. The perfume was astoundingly opulent, a triple dose of spices and woods that proved addictive. I wore it with passion, and even today the glamorous, snuggly scent reminds me of crackling fireplaces, après-ski evenings, and snow-capped mountains rising in the distance.

Isn't it interesting the memories a perfume can conjure? It's true; our sense of smell is a powerful, often unconscious, trigger for memories—even those long-buried.

Scent Type: Spicy-Woody Oriental
Top Notes: Plum, hesperides, clove, coriander, pepper, bay leaf
Heart Notes: Jasmine, rose, carnation, lily of the valley, cinnamon, peach, orris
Base Notes: Sandalwood, vetiver, myrrh, opopanax, labdanum, benzoin, benjamin, castoreum, amber, incense, musk, patchouli, tolu

Who's Worn It
Salma Hayek, Emily Blunt, Hilary Duff, Heidi Klum, Tanya Tucker, Jerry Hall, Martine McCutcheon, Gisele Bundchen

Introduced: 1977

***

Oscar

Oscar de la Renta

In 1978, couturier Oscar de la Renta enchanted the world with his first fragrance foray. His signature scent, created by perfumer Jean-Louis Sieuzac, is an intensely

Vintage Perfumes

feminine floral Oriental perfume which includes a rich white floral bouquet bursting with tuberose, jasmine, and orange blossom.

De la Renta took his inspiration from his mother's flower garden in which grew the fragrant white flowers of his native country, the Dominican Republic. The finale is a quietly sensual blend of sandalwood, amber, and myrrh. Excellent for daytime, exquisite for evening. Soft, subtle, sweet, and sophisticated.

The fragrance is featured in a curved glass flacon from bottle designer Serge Mansau and capped with a frosted glass flower with a dewdrop nestled among the petals. The fragrance garnered a pair of 1978 Fragrance Foundation FiFi Awards and earned a coveted spot in the FiFi US Hall of Fame.

Oscar de la Renta's signature fragrance: A polished thoroughbred, romantically inclined.

Jan's Note: Ah, the memories this perfume holds for me…Oscar was one of the first perfumes I represented when I entered the perfume industry. What memories do you have that are conjured by perfume?

Scent Type: Floral Oriental
Top Notes: Orange blossom, coriander, cascarilla, basil, peach, gardenia
Heart Notes: Jasmine, tuberose, ylang-ylang, May rose, lavender, orchid
Base Notes: Clove, sandalwood, amber, myrrh, lavender, patchouli, opopanax

Who's Worn It
Princess Margaret, Sharon Stone, Hillary Clinton, Martine McCutcheon

Introduced: 1978

***

Paloma Picasso Mon Parfum
Paloma Picasso

From internationally acclaimed designer Paloma Picasso comes a signature fragrance as worldly, dramatic, and elegant as its creator. She states: "It is a fragrance for women, not girls. It is sophisticated, not naive or innocent." She calls it "jewelry for the senses."

The lush, slightly smoky chypre perfume created by Francis Bocris begins with brisk citrus and fresh green notes. It dissolves into rich jeweled notes of jasmine and Bulgarian rose which are poised against layers of patchouli and oakmoss. Presented in a flawless crystal ball, the perfume is wreathed by frosted French glass or a plastic casing, depending on the packaging, which is designed in Paloma's signature Florentine red and black.

As the daughter of artist Pablo Picasso and Francoise Gilot, Paloma Picasso was born into a world of creativity. She was christened Paloma, meaning "dove" in Spanish, after her father's dove which was the symbol of the 1949 Peace Congress. She expressed her artistic genius in myriad ways, from her jewelry designs for Tiffany to her china and crystal creations for Villeroy & Boch.

She says: "As jewelry can please the eye and the hand, so fragrance can please the senses...revealing new sensory delights layer by layer. It is an intimate ornament that becomes part of your identity...a part of the mosaic of your life." Her philosophy is evident in her signature fragrance, a jewel in itself.

Jan's Note: Not long ago a friend wore a perfume that was so amazing on her—and so familiar, although I couldn't place it. Turns out it was Mon Parfum, as unapologetically lush and smoky as ever. If you loved it once and haven't tried it in a while, it's definitely worth a revisit.

Scent Type: Chypre – Floral
Top Notes: Bergamot, neroli, lemon, ambrette
Heart Notes: Jasmine, Bulgarian rose, ylang-ylang, coriander, clove
Base Notes: Patchouli, vetiver, sandalwood, oakmoss, moss, amber

Introduced: 1984

***

Paris
Yves Saint Laurent

In this magnificent rose bouquet, Yves Saint Laurent and perfumer Sophia Grojsman captured the very essence of the grand city of Paris.

Paris is a profuse bundle of flowers with rich sweet rose top notes and heady floral heart notes set against warm woods and moss. An abundance of femininity sparkles in its spirit and soul. Paris is an extravagant, radiant fragrance for the fearless romantic-at-heart. One of the most magnificent rose-centered perfumes ever created, Paris is a complete rose immersion.

Think of Paris in the springtime, the Place Vendôme, the rue de Rivoli, the Louvre, the Musee D'Orsay. Fittingly, Paris is packaged in rose petal pink and chic jet black.

Vintage Perfumes

Jan's Note: Paris is a truly legendary rose perfume for rose aficionados created by the incomparable Sophia Grojsman, a perfumer known for her exquisite compositions. Paris is the bold interpretation of a thousand roses bursting from budded confines under sunny spring skies. In Paris, of course.

Scent Type: Floral
Top Notes: Rose petals, orange blossom, mimosa, cassia, hawthorn, nasturtium, bergamot, greens, hyacinth
Heart Notes: Rose, violet leaves, jasmine, orris, ylang-ylang, lily of the valley, lily, linden blossom
Base Notes: Sandalwood, amber, musk, moss, iris, cedarwood, heliotrope

Who's Worn It
Lynn Wyatt

Introduced: 1984

***

Parure
Guerlain

Parure is a fragrant jewel, a sophisticated perfume from fifth-generation Guerlain perfumer Jean-Paul Guerlain who created Parure in honor of his mother, Lily Guerlain.

An unaffected blend of chypre, fruit, and floral notes

results in a lightly balanced, elegant perfume. Distinctly feminine, Guerlain says Parure is "for an aesthetic, discerning woman, constantly in search of quality and truth." Parure is French for "adornment," referring to precious luxuries, but it also refers to a suite, or set of jewelry.

Whereas Guerlain created Chamade for the modern liberated woman, and Chant d'Arômes for youthful innocence, Parure was designed for the woman who is at ease with herself and appreciates the luxuries her life holds.

Scent Type: Chypre - Floral
Top Notes: Plum, bergamot, fruits, hesperides, greens
Heart Notes: Rose, lilac, jasmine, lily of the valley, jonquil, narcissus, orris
Base Notes: Oakmoss, patchouli, spices, amber, leather

Who's Worn It
Lily Guerlain, Wendy Wasserstein

Introduced: 1975

***

Vintage Perfumes

Passion

Annick Goutal

Two years in the making, this rich, sensual fragrance was developed in Grasse, France by Annick Goutal. Not to be confused with her own Gardénia Passion, nor with Elizabeth Taylor's Passion.

Passion is a heady combination of rich white flowers balanced by tenacious vanilla. The effect is languorous, a tropical island evening with warm, flower-laden air.

A long-lasting, intensely feminine fragrance, Passion is appropriately named according to the Victorian language of flowers. White jasmine meant amiability, yellow jasmine conveyed grace and elegance, while Spanish jasmine denoted sensuality. And tuberose? Dangerous pleasures. Passion is a lively fragrance with a dangerous abundance of significant florals.

Scent Type: Floral
Top Notes: Ylang-ylang
Heart Notes: Jasmine, tuberose, ylang-ylang
Base Notes: Vanilla

Who's Worn It
Princess Caroline of Monaco, Sylvie Vartan, Ali MacGraw

Introduced: 1986

Pavlova
Payot

A tender classic floral, Pavlova was created in honor of the glorious Russian prima ballerina Anna Pavlova who lived from 1885 to 1931. Fragrance is a beautiful part of Russian ballet history, and Pavlova is a tribute to the art.

Legend has it that in ballets of yore each ballerina was assigned a perfume to be worn with extravagance on the body and hair. Thus, the ballet was an experience not only in vision and sound but also in smell. Patrons could close their eyes and imagine gliding through a flower garden so sweet was the symphony of fragrance from the dancers. Russian ballet impresario and founder of the Ballet Russes, Sergei Diaghilev, practiced this, and fellow Russian-born choreographer George Balanchine continued the tradition with the American Ballet Theater in New York City which he founded in 1933.

Pavlova is presented in dramatic black flacons enhanced by delicate pink flowers that entwine the bottles. Others are of clear glass featuring a graceful swan. Long after the fragrance is finished, the bottles will beautify any dressing table. They are as lovely as the fragrance, a romantic, fresh floral scent.

Jan's Note: Ballet has always been dear to my heart. My mother studied ballet under Alexander Kotchetovsky, a

Vintage Perfumes

Diaghilev ballet dancer and Bolshoi alumnus who also trained actor Gene Kelly in dance. My ballet training began when I was young, and my perfume of choice was often Pavlova. Even today, this perfume will whisk me backstage before a ballet performance.

Scent Type: Floral
Top Notes: Hyacinth, bergamot, galbanum, black currant bud
Heart Notes: Rose, jasmine, tuberose, orchid, narcissus, orris
Base Notes: Sandalwood, musk, amber, cedarwood, benzoin, moss

Who's Worn It
Ballerina Anna Pavlova

Introduced: 1922

***

Polo
Ralph Lauren

Who would have thought to see Polo in a vintage perfume guide? And yet, here it is—at the time of writing, this fragrance is closing in on forty years old. For many men, it was their first fragrance. Their father or grandfather might have worn Old Spice, so Polo was a distinct change of pace for the younger generation. American designer Ralph Lauren put a brilliant lifestyle marketing campaign behind it, and the rest is history.

Upon its debut, Polo quickly achieved superstar status. Packaged in the familiar hunter green and gold bottle, Polo is a crisp chypre formula created by perfumer Carlos Benaïm that zips open on a green herbal note. The heart holds masculine impressions of leather and tobacco while the oakmoss and patchouli blend results in a classic chypre combination.

At once dry and smoky and sweet, Polo is a well-balanced composition that deserves its place in history. Polo is in the FiFi Hall of Fame, a recognition bestowed by The Fragrance Foundation.

Scent Type: Chypre
Top Notes: Basil, chamomile
Heart Notes: Leather, tobacco
Base Notes: Oakmoss, patchouli

Introduced: 1978

***

Vintage Perfumes

Pour Une Femme
Caron

Pure femininity is the hallmark of Pour Une Femme de Caron, meaning "for a woman," a luminous floral orchestration originally created in 1942.

Caron founding perfumer Ernest Daltroff employed his classic soft rose bouquet sweetening it with raspberry and green mandarin. Amber and musk enrich the finale with quiet opulence. Perfumer Richard Fraysse recreated this perfume. The main impression is of rose and woods.

Pour Une Femme is a romantic, radiant fragrance with a nostalgic nature. The bottle features curvaceous lines fashioned after the female torso.

Scent Type: Powdery Floral
Top Notes: Mandarin, raspberry
Heart Notes: Jasmine, rose, Egyptian Rose
Base Notes: Amber, musk

Introduced: 1942
***

Private Collection
Estée Lauder

Private Collection is an enthralling green-themed composition that was Estée Lauder's private perfume.

Rich and elegant, this 1973 classic is a mélange of rose, galbanum, and patchouli. A perennial statement of feminine glamour, Private Collection was also a favorite of Grace Kelly, Her Serene Highness Princess Grace of Monaco.

Lauder often tested a variety of scents in progress and naturally had a cache of personal favorites. Once when asked what scent she was wearing, Lauder replied that it was from her private collection. Soon, customers began asking for "private collection" at Lauder counters. Thus was born Private Collection. Whether this was clever marketing or the real truth, the fragrance remains a classic.

Jan's Note: Private Collection is an astute balance between white-glove femininity and corner-office CEO, which seems to mirror Estée Lauder's position, circa 1973. A remarkable achievement for a perfume of that era.

Scent Type: Chypre – Green
Top Notes: Greens, hyacinth, citrus
Heart Notes: Jasmine, narcissus, rose, pine, reseda
Base Notes: Oakmoss, cedarwood, amber, musk

Vintage Perfumes

Who's Worn It
Princess Grace of Monaco

Introduced: 1973

***

Que sais-je?
Jean Patou

Que sais-je? is the second of Jean Patou's fragrant 1925 love trilogy, which also included Amour Amour and Adieu Sagesse. It was inspired by the moment when the will hesitates.

Meaning "What do I know?," Que sais-je? is a light, flowery chypre blend. Patou suggested this fragrance for fair-skinned blond women, but anyone can enjoy this fresh composition which was reformulated by Jean Kerléo, the in-house master perfumer for Jean Patou. It was originally created by master perfumer Henri Alméras.

Pronounce it "Kuh se-zhe."

Scent Type: Chypre – Fruity
Top Notes: Peach, apricot, orange blossom
Heart Notes: Jasmine, rose, carnation, iris
Base Notes: Oakmoss, patchouli

Who's Worn It
Constance Bennett, Josephine Baker

Introduced: 1925

***

Quelques Fleurs L'Original
Houbigant

One of the most important fragrances in history, Quelques Fleurs was the first true multi-floral composition, reportedly utilizing 313 different floral essences. Its development changed the approach to perfumery in the early 1900s, from subtle single florals to radiant multi-floral bouquets, and firmly established Paris as the foremost city of perfumery.

In 1987, Houbigant responded to consumer requests and reintroduced the fragrance which is a devastatingly feminine scent, classic and sophisticated, and evocative of sun-drenched gardens brimming with intoxicating flowers. Freshened with greens and warmed with ambery woods, the perfume is a beautifully balanced bouquet.

Jan's Note: Quelques Fleurs L'Original is a lovely reminder of the beauty of La Belle Époque. Even the most legendary actress of the era, Sarah Bernhardt (known as the Divine Sarah in her day), was a devoted fan of ravishing perfume.

Vintage Perfumes

Scent Type: Floral
Top Notes: Greens, bergamot, orange blossom, lemon, tarragon
Heart Notes: Rose, jasmine, tuberose, lily of the valley, ylang-ylang, carnation, heliotrope, orchid, orris
Base Notes: Sandalwood, oakmoss, amber, musk, tonka bean, civet

Who's Worn It
Daisy Fuentes, Sarah Bernhardt, Dita Von Teese, Josette Banzet the Marquise de Bruyenne, Kelly Rowland, Ginnifer Goodwin, Nicole Richie

Introduced: 1912
***

Rive Gauche
Yves Saint Laurent

From designer Yves Saint Laurent, Rive Gauche is a profusion of rose and delicate, sweet white flowers, placed against a backdrop of woods and moss, all briskly introduced with ephemeral aldehydic notes. Rive Gauche is Paris, circa 1969.

Perfumer Jacques Polge, who went on to work for Chanel as their in-house perfumer, created Rive Gauche which many industry professionals consider one of the finest floral aldehyde, or powdery floral, perfumes ever created. It was recreated in 2003 by perfumer Jacques Hy and Daniela Andrier, and the result is similar, yet lighter and fresher.

Rive Gauche has a pleasing modern beat. Look for Rive Gauche in the traditional midnight blue-and-black ribbed aluminum bottle.

Jan's Note: I once worked for Yves Saint Laurent, and as a result, Rive Gauche, Opium, and Paris are forever imprinted on my olfactory memory. Rive Gauche always reminded me of an independent, innovative woman who was confident in her abilities and ready to take on the world.

Rive Gauche means "Left Bank" in French, and was always the traditional bohemian Paris haunt of writers, artists, and philosophers, such as Colette, Henry Miller, Anais Nin, Gertrude Stein, Alice B. Toklas, Edith Wharton, Pablo Picasso, Henri Matisse, Jean-Paul Sartre, Ernest Hemingway, F. Scott Fitzgerald, and so many more...

Scent Type: Powdery Floral
Top Notes: Aldehydes, bergamot, greens, peach
Heart Notes: Magnolia, jasmine, gardenia, geranium, iris, ylang-ylang, rose, lily of the valley
Base Notes: Mysore sandalwood, Haitian vetiver, tonka bean, musk, moss, amber

Who's Worn It
Katherine Hepburn, Joanna Lumley, Barbara Hutton

Vintage Perfumes

Introduced: 1969

***

Rose Absolue
Annick Goutal

An international cornucopia of roses was gathered for this brilliant, fragrant exaltation from Annick Goutal. It is a superbly feminine fragrance celebrating the rose, the queen of flowers.

The scent of the rose is one of nature's most powerfully sensual aromas, and the rose is one of the most coveted flowers in history. In old Persia, the Sultan slept on a mattress filled with rose petals. Fountains of rose water adorned tables at feasts, and rose petals were often strewn among party guests. In the Victorian language of flowers, roses are the symbol of love. White roses represent purity and spiritual love; red roses mean true love; cabbage roses are ambassadors of love; a single rose denotes simplicity; burgundy roses mean unconscious beauty. But beware the yellow rose, for it represents decreasing love and infidelity.

Rose Absolue is made of high quality roses, including the May rose, or rose de mai, Damascena, Bulgarian, Egyptian, and Moroccan. Each one of these roses has a slightly different scent, so when blended, the resulting rose aroma is rich and full-bodied. Goutal envisioned Rose Absolue as a perfume that could be worn by itself or blended with others in her line. Most all Goutal perfumes are made to be worn alone or layered with others in the line.

Jan's Note: One of my favorite combinations is Rose Absolue with Goutal's Eau d'Hadrien. Try layering these two on the skin by applying Rose Absolue first followed by Eau d'Hadrien. While Rose Absolue is lovely by itself, I enjoy the freshness that Eau d'Hadrien brings to the mix by adding a dollop of sunshine and a warm wooded finish with a slight green accent.

Scent Type: Floral
Notes: May rose, Turkish rose, Bulgarian rose, Damascus rose, Egyptian rose, Moroccan rose

Introduced: 1986

***

Royal Secret
Germaine Monteil

Germaine Monteil introduced Royal Secret in 1935 at a time when royal families still had secrets. The 1930s were the height of fascination with all things from the Orient of old, and Royal Secret reflects this with its eastern composition.

The fiery creation opens with fresh citrus notes then combines a classic French heart of jasmine and rose with exotic base notes of sandalwood, musk, and myrrh.

Royal Secret...as rich and engaging as ever.

Scent Type: Spicy-Woody Oriental
Top Notes: Citrus, African orange
Heart Notes: Bulgarian rose, jasmine
Base Notes: Sandalwood, musk, myrrh

Introduced: 1935

***

Shalimar
Guerlain

Shalimar is an intoxicating yet subtly sensuous blend that has endured for more than sixty-five years. With a long-lasting base of spices and aromatic woods, it became the archetype for Oriental blends. A highly distinctive and dramatic fragrance, it was designed for the woman who is sensual, sophisticated and uninhibited...another grand entrance-making perfume from Guerlain.

A 1925 composition, Shalimar is reflective of its period, of a cosmopolitan Paris in the midst of celebration after World War I, of the Roaring Twenties, of exhilaration and new life. This attitude is mirrored in the zesty citrus top notes. Heady florals flow into a spicy base that is particularly rich in vanilla, incense, and sandalwood.

In creating Shalimar, Jacques Guerlain was inspired by a love story told to him by a Maharajah visiting Paris. The

Guerlain company shared the story with us:

> More than 300 years ago, Shah Jahan succeeded to the throne of his father, Jahangir, and became the third Mogul Emperor of India.
>
> Jahan loved only one woman. Her name was Mumtaz Mahal.
>
> Some say he loved her unto madness, that she was not his wife but his fever. Victories, empires and riches were dust as compared to her...in his eyes, she alone was the balm that made life bearable.
>
> When she died, Jahan's hair turned white. He would burst into tears at the mention of her name. In her memory, he built one of the world's greatest wonders–the Taj Mahal at Agra.
>
> But the Taj Mahal is only an empty monument. While Mumtaz was alive, Jahan created a series of gardens for her at Lahore, gardens the like of which had never been seen before. He called them the gardens of Shalimar, the Sanskrit word meaning "abode of love."
>
> From every corner of the Earth, the most fragrant and delicate blossoms were brought. Deep pools were built with crystal fountains and terraces paved in marble. The rarest birds were summoned to sing here and lanterns were hung to rival the stars. In the gardens of Shalimar the lovers were truly happy, and Mumtaz bore fourteen children to her beloved Jahan.

Vintage Perfumes

Jacques Guerlain decided that the perfume should be called Shalimar, not Taj Mahal, because, you see, Taj Mahal marks the end of the story, and this love story can never end.

The flacon was designed by Raymond Guerlain and is also a reminder of the fountains in the gardens of Shalimar. The ornamental stopper in sapphire blue evokes the flow of the fountains' water.

Voluptuous and enveloping, Shalimar is a fragrance of eternal romance.

Jan's Note: I grew up with Shalimar on the arms of my mother when she hugged me before bedtime. And so, when I was in my early teens, I thought Shalimar a dowdy, old lady fragrance, as a teenager might. Imagine my surprise a few years later when I unknowingly encountered it at a party. The most intriguing, elegant woman in the room wore a fascinating perfume on which men were complimenting her. *I knew that aroma,* I thought, *but what is it?* "Do you mind if I ask what you're wearing?" I asked. She confided, "Shalimar." True elegance is timeless.

A sensual delight with a dichotomy of dry and sweet, Shalimar is the original gourmand aroma with a plush vanilla note, as tactile as velvet or the softest silk lining.

JAN MORAN

Scent Type: Vanilla-Ambery Oriental
Top Notes: Bergamot, lemon, hesperides
Heart Notes: Jasmine, iris, rose, patchouli, vetiver
Base Notes: Vanilla, incense, opopanax, sandalwood, musk, civet, ambergris, leather

Who's Worn It
Rita Hayworth, Gina Lollobrigida, Diane Sawyer, Brooke Shields, Rita Hayworth, Dionne Warwick, Britt Ekland, Joan Collins, Lisa Hartman, Shirley McClaine, and my mother, Jeanne Hollenbeck

Introduced: 1925

***

Sikkim
Lancôme

The former kingdom of Sikkim stretches high into the Himalayan mountains of India's northwest region. Isolated from the outside world, Sikkim is steeped in ancient traditions. The French firm of Lancôme pays tribute to Sikkim with a nostalgic fragrance.

With its aura of mystery, Sikkim is a rich arrangement of patchouli, amber, and vanilla while rose adds an element of romance. Quietly alluring, Sikkim is a perfume suited for seduction. Lancôme says it is "For a woman destined to achieve her dreams."

Vintage Perfumes

Jan's Note: Years ago I visited the bazaars in Mumbai, and lodged in my olfactory memory is the rich aromatic mélange of fresh-cut flowers, Eastern spices, and hand-tooled leather. The first time I tested Sikkim, I closed my eyes, and it was as if I'd been teleported to an Indian bazaar. Lush, silky, seductive. A little hard to find, but certainly worth it.

Scent Type: Floral Oriental
Top Notes: Bergamot
Heart Notes: Jasmine, rose
Base Notes: Leather, patchouli, vanilla, amber

Introduced: 1971

***

Soir de Paris (Evening in Paris)
Bourjois

In 1928, legendary perfumer Ernest Beaux, who created Chanel No. 5, originated another beloved perfume, Soir de Paris. It was also marketed as Evening in Paris in English-speaking markets. In 1969, Soir de Paris was discontinued.

Fast forward to 1992 when perfumers Jacques Polge and Francois Demarchy recreated the classic fragrance. The modern version features a fresh opening accord of apricot and peach, which segues to a vibrant rose-jasmine heart, and a powdery iris-sandalwood finale.

Soir de Paris is a long-lasting, little-black-dress-and-pearls perfume and is still ensconced in bottles of magnetic midnight blue.

Jan's Note: In a tiny antique shop in Palm Springs, I discovered a dusty brown box on a lower shelf. When I opened it, there lay a gift set of Soir de Paris, its sapphire bottles undimmed by time. Though the perfume has turned a bit, I still cherish this perfume from my childhood.

Scent Type: Floral
Top Notes: Apricot, bergamot, violet leaves
Heart Notes: Rose, jasmine, lily of the valley, ylang-ylang, orris
Base Notes: Peach, amber, sandalwood, vanilla

Introduced: 1928

***

Sous Le Vent
Guerlain

Originally created in 1933, Jacques Guerlain's Sous Le Vent combines Greta Garbo's cool elegance with Jean Harlow's irresistible charm. With the reissue (in 2006) of Sous Le Vent (pronounced 'soo luh vahn'), Guerlain allows a glimpse into its magnificent archives and its illustrious past.

The vivacious sparkle of bergamot, lavender, and tarragon sets the stage for a sumptuous heart of iris and jasmine which is lifted with fresh green notes. Dry woods juxtapose the scent's airy green nature in this chypre, or mossy-woody fragrance. Enjoy the timeless seduction of this vintage jewel.

"With perfumes, it is impossible to be too audacious. At Guerlain, the emphasis has always been placed on raw materials and preserving a spirit of independence from fashion's dictates." House of Guerlain

Scent Type: Mossy-Woody
Notes: Jasmine, Lavender, Ylang-Ylang, Green Notes

Who's Worn It
Josephine Baker

Introduced: 1933

***

Spanish Leather
Geo. F. Trumper

More than a century has passed since Spanish Leather was created in Great Britain, but the company of Geo. F. Trumper still remain true to the artistic vision of the original Spanish Leather.

Spanish Leather is a mélange of spicy clove and the resinous sweetness of patchouli—a dark, rich combination that conjures images of the exotic travels of yesteryear. A heart of rose melds the elements and endows the fragrance with a romantic overture.

Spanish Leather is for men with a romantic soul. A fine example of turn-of-the-century British perfumery for gentlemen.

Jan's Note: When I was writing my historical novel, *Scent of Triumph*, I searched for fragrance that a well-groomed, well-traveled man of the British Empire might wear in 1939. Closing my eyes, I led my devastatingly handsome male character, Jonathan Newell-Grey, through gentlemen's shops in Mayfair. Soon we came to number 9 Curzon Street where Geo. F. Trumper, Gentlemen's Barber, is located, not far from the Ritz Hotel.

I had walked these lanes when I stayed at Brown's Hotel with my son, so everything was still fresh in my mind. As I ran through the fragrances, auditioning them for Jon, I must admit that Bay Rum was close, but Spanish Leather won out. With its rich, intriguing blend of rose, spice, and woods, it has the heart of a lover and the soul of an adventurer.

Scent Type: Spicy-Woody Oriental
Notes: Musk, patchouli, clove, rose

Who's Worn It
Jonathan Newell-Grey

Vintage Perfumes

Introduced: 1902

***

Tabac Blond
Caron

From 1919, Tabac Blond is a Caron classic dedicated to liberated women. French for "blond tobacco," Caron's founding perfumer, Ernest Daltroff, created this provocative dry wooded fragrance with women who smoked in mind. Allied soldiers' cigarettes inspired his rich impressions of tobacco and leather, woven with powdery iris and earthy vetiver, and rendered creamy with amber and vanilla—a Caron signature flourish.

Favored by actress Marlene Dietrich, vintage Tabac Blond is glamorous and seductive, a refined scent reminiscent of crisp autumn leaves, smoldering fireplaces, and worn leather sofas. For women—and men—who savor the unusual, for those with the audacity to defy convention.

Jan's Note: The original Tabac Blond was dark, smoky, dry, and gorgeous. One was immediately whisked to that period of time in Europe wedged between the end of World War I and the Depression. The Roaring Twenties were a time to grasp the life that had ebbed away for many lost in the war, and Tabac Blond reflected this time of daring.

However, recent regulations on perfumery ingredients

have forced an edit for many vintage fragrances. While some are virtually unchanged, others received a more drastic reformulation. Today's Tabac Blond has less of its original dry smoky character and has more emphasis on carnation, though the woods are still present. Green accents have been added, and though not as va-va-vivacious as it once was, it's still enough to turn heads.

As a side note, in the early 1900s vintage Tabac Blond had such an *avant-garde* following that it was another perfume I chose for a character in my novel, *Scent of Triumph*. How I wish it still existed in its vintage form…

Scent Type: Woody
Notes: Leather, patchouli, vanilla, amber, iris, vetiver, musk, carnation, ylang-ylang

Who's Worn It
Marlene Dietrich

Introduced: 1919

***

Vanille (Vanille Passion)
Comptoir Sud Pacifique

Vanille Passion is a vanilla-infused gourmet treat. This 1978 fragrance proved so popular it launched the French firm of Comptoir Sud Pacifique. Also known simply as

Vanille, it may be worn alone or layered with other fragrances in the firm's line.

The sweet beguiling essence of vanilla is pure intoxication. It's a sweet, languorous combination of culinary sensuality. Vanilla is harvested from the seed pods of the vanilla orchid plant. Some of the world's best vanilla comes from Madagascar, an Indian Ocean island.

Though a newer fragrance, Comptoir Sud Pacifique's Vanille Abricot is also worth trying and is one of the company's perennial bestsellers. Pair these island travel scents with sandals and sunglasses, and then pack your bags and say *adieu*.

Jan's Note: Vanille Passion blooms in the moist warmth of the islands. Simple, sweet, and sexy, it's one of my must-have perfumes for beach holidays.

Scent Type: Vanilla-Amber Oriental
Top Notes: Tahitian Vanilla
Heart Notes: Vanilla bean
Base Notes: Vanilla

Who's Worn It
Sienna Miller

Introduced: 1978

***

JAN MORAN

Vent Vert
Balmain

Created by renowned perfumer Germaine Cellier for Paris couturier Pierre Balmain, Vent Vert is a green floral fragrance that has undergone recent formula renovations. The original fragrance was a remarkable feat of vibrant galbanum, green and ripe as early spring, lush with the scent of a meadow blanketed with a rainbow of wildflowers, tender shoots of emerald grass, and damp, mossy earth underneath.

Vent Vert is French for "green breeze," and in Cellier's hands, it was a bold spring wind that paved the way for many green fragrances of today.

Jan's Note: Due to scarcity of ingredients and changing regulations, Vent Vert has been reformulated on at least two occasions. The intensity had been toned down, as long-time wearers might notice. Someday, perhaps, the incandescent brilliance might surface again, but in the meantime, the current Vent Vert is a lighter, fresh version of the marvelous original, and more in tune with modern tastes.

Scent Type: Floral – Green
Top Notes: Greens, orange blossom, lemon, lime, basil
Heart Notes: Galbanum, lily of the valley, freesia, hyacinth, rose, tagetes, ylang-ylang, violet
Base Notes: Oakmoss, sandalwood, sage, iris, amber, musk

Vintage Perfumes

Who's Worn It
Brigitte Bardot

Introduced: 1947

***

Vetiver
Guerlain

Guerlain is well known for its wide array of fragrances for women and men. From the unisex fougère Jicky to the memorable Mitsouko and Shalimar for women, Guerlain has proved its mastery of the art of perfume over several generations.

Vetiver, like most Guerlain fragrances, began with an inspiration. The story is told of Jean-Paul Guerlain, then a young perfumer, who happened upon a country squire who had just left his estate. A woody green aroma clung to his clothes mingled with the smoky sweetness of tobacco. Guerlain's nose surely tingled with excitement. The result is a woody green blend, freshened with citrus, spiked with tobacco and spice, smoothed and rounded with tonka bean.

Derived from a woody root, vetiver is a tenacious essential oil. Although Vetiver was made for men, women gravitate toward it, too, and their skin chemistry evokes a subtle difference. Vetiver is a classic formula, understated and refined, a scent of casual ease.

Jan's Note: On a trip to Normandy, I once stayed at a grand country home. In the salon in front of an open window stood a carved vetiver screen, its woody-green scent dispersed through the room with each billow of hand-made lace curtains. Sweet pipe tobacco hung in the air, offset by the scent of surrounding evergreens—the entire effect was incredibly reminiscent of Guerlain's Vetiver.

Scent Type: Chypre
Top Notes: Citrus
Heart Notes: Vetiver, spices
Base Notes: Tobacco, sandalwood, tonka bean

Who's Worn It
Jodi Foster, Naomi Campbell, Anne Bass, Andy Garcia, Harrison Ford, Paul McCartney, Arnold Schwarzenegger, John Fairchild, Michael Caine, Peter Sellers

Introduced: 1959

***

Visa

Robert Piguet

Robert Piguet was one of the most influential couturiers in Paris in the 1930s and during World War II. For many years, his salon in Paris featured his tasteful daytime collections as well as flamboyant evening wear. Young

Vintage Perfumes

designers such as Hubert de Givenchy and Pierre Balmain studied under him, learning their craft. And then came World War II. Piguet continued working, refusing to succumb to pressures to move his salon to Berlin and in the process, retaining employment for hundreds who worked directly or indirectly for him.

The original Visa was created by perfumer Jean Carles (some credit Germaine Cellier, but records appear to indicate Jean Carles), who also blended Tabu. In fact, these were quite similar in nature: heady Oriental perfumes, dark and voluptuous, mysterious and memorable.

However, times change, and so do vintage perfumes. The new edition, created by Aurelién Guichard, is far different, yet immensely fine. The smooth, succulent note of peach sets the stage for a rich floral heart of rose and ylang-ylang. A leathery-woody accord is the grand finale, which lingers on the skin with a sense of vintage mystery.

Scent Type: Chypre
Top Notes: Bergamot, pear, ylang-ylang, violet leaves, mandarin
Heart Notes: Rose, peach, immortelle, orange flower absolute
Base Notes: Sandalwood, leather, patchouli, moss, vetiver, vanilla

Introduced: 1947

Vol de Nuit
Guerlain

Another timeless classic from Jacques Guerlain, Vol de Nuit is a warm vanilla-infused perfume designed for the elusive, assertive woman.

Vol de Nuit, French for "night flight," is presented in a dramatic, gold-colored amber bottle molded in the shape of French Air Force wings. Vol de Nuit was created in homage to the daring aviators of the 1920s and named after the Antoine de Saint-Exupéry novel, *Vol de Nuit*, about nighttime mail flights to South America. Saint-Exupéry, also an avid aviator, was the author of many works, including *Le Petit Prince*.

Blended of spice, galbanum, amber, and vanilla, Vol de Nuit reflects the pure, unvarnished essence of adventure, the spirit of exploration, and the radiance of independence. With a preponderance of rich raw ingredients, lightly woven, it has a natural heartthrob of exotic sensuality. This is the audacious, unadulterated aroma of the 1930s, a time of adventure into the wild unknown.

Jan's Note: Vol de Nuit is still one of the most marvelous vintage perfumes around. If you love vanilla and amber, you must try Vol de Nuit. I have a vintage bottle, and it's remarkably similar to the current edition; the difference is most likely in the aging as volatile citrus notes tend to

Vintage Perfumes

dissipate over time in perfumes. One whiff and I'm immediately transported to a red-cushioned booth in a little vintage jazz club in Paris...

Scent Type: Vanilla-Ambery Oriental
Top Notes: Orange, mandarin, lemon, bergamot, orange blossom
Heart Notes: Jonquil, aldehydes, galbanum
Base Notes: Vanilla, spices, oakmoss, sandalwood, orris, musk

Who's Worn It
Claudette Colbert, Katherine Hepburn, Barbra Streisand, Michelle Pfeiffer, Diana Rigg, Carla Bruni

Introduced: 1933

***

White Linen
Estée Lauder

Estée Lauder was searching for the fragrant embodiment of white linen, a scentthat was clean, crisp, and classic. She and fragrance legend Sophia Grojsman achieved this in the development of White Linen, the fragrance.

White Linen is a fragrance with a brightly polished demeanor. Brisk aldehydic top notes are shower-fresh and slightly soapy. A delicate rose-infused floral bouquet benefits from the green accent of hyacinth and lily of the valley. The scent lingers with warm, comfortable-as-cotton background notes. The effect is one of understated sophistication, the epitome of relaxed American style.

Jan's Note: White Linen is often a surprise to people who like powdery aldehydic florals, such as Chanel No. 5 or Chanel No. 22, or even Red by Giorgio. Sophia Grojsman is a genius in perfumery and has been honored by the American Society of Perfumers for her lifetime achievements. She also created Trésor, Paris, and Beautiful among many other perfumes, plus, her work with roses is nothing short of magical. If you haven't tried White Linen, put it on your list. It's a well-priced delight.

Scent Type: Powdery Floral
Top Notes: Jasmine, Bulgarian rose, aldehydes, lily of the valley
Heart Notes: Hyacinth, jasmine, lily of the valley, violet, iris (orris)
Base Notes: Oakmoss, vetiver

Introduced: 1978
***

Vintage Perfumes

White Shoulders
Elizabeth Arden

White Shoulders is an enduring floral as charming today as when it was introduced. The predominant note is tuberose, sweet, delicate, and feminine with a powdery soft finish. Originally produced by Evyan, the perfume is currently distributed by Elizabeth Arden (though distribution companies frequently trade lines).

Legend has it that White Shoulders was inspired by a baron's love for a woman with exquisite porcelain shoulders, the woman whose cameo still embellishes each pink package.

White Shoulders whispers of a bygone era, of daring low-cut ball gowns, billowing satin, and rustling taffeta. An intoxicating scent, it continues to enchant each new generation.

Jan's Note: I'm sure I'm not the only person who associates White Shoulders with a beloved grandmother. It always brings a little smile to my lips…

Scent Type: Floral
Top Notes: Neroli, tuberose, aldehydes
Heart Notes: Gardenia, jasmine, orris, lily of the valley, rose, lilac
Base Notes: Sandalwood, amber, musk, oakmoss

JAN MORAN

Who's Worn It
Barbara Bush

Introduced: 1935

***

Wind Song
Matchabelli

Memories abound in Wind Song, the 1952 classic floral fragrance by Prince George Matchabelli, the Italian prince of the Belle Époque era who gave the world a collection of fine fragrances blended by perfumer Ernest Shiftan in remembrance.

Mandarin and leafy greens comprise Wind Song's fresh opening. Jasmine and ylang-ylang, spiced with sweet clove, form a graceful heart while sandalwood, musk, and amber provide a silky, powdery finish.

Embodying 1950s femininity, Wind Song remains a sentimental favorite. Although the formula has been changed from the original, this is still a pleasant fragrance at an affordable price.

Scent Type: Powdery Floral
Top Notes: Bergamot, lily of the valley
Heart Notes: Jasmine, rose
Base Notes: Sandalwood

Vintage Perfumes

Introduced: 1952

***

Y

Yves Saint Laurent

Y was the first fragrance introduced by couturier Yves Saint Laurent. Completely different from his later flamboyant creations, Opium and Paris, Y is a light fragrance, delicate, feminine, and subtle.

Perfumers Jacques Bercia and Michel Hy worked together to create this classic perfume. It's a peach-infused chypre blend with a vivid green note drawn of gardenia, galbanum, and oakmoss. Y is a fresh, modern fragrance for forward-thinking souls. Well, Y not?

Jan's Note: It's easy to see the influence of early 1960s modernity in this departure from classic vintage perfumes of the past. In the 1960s world of *Mad Men* style, Y would have appealed to Don Draper's second wife, Megan, while first wife Betty would have worn Miss Dior.

Y is a vintage fragrance of style, not passing fashion. Yves Saint Laurent said it best: "Fashions fade, style is eternal."

Scent Type: Chypre
Top Notes: Greens, aldehydes, peach, gardenia, honeysuckle, galbanum
Heart Notes: Bulgarian rose, jasmine, tuberose, ylang-ylang, orris, hyacinth
Base Notes: Oakmoss, amber, patchouli, sandalwood, vetiver, civet, benzoin, styrax

Introduced: 1964

***

Youth Dew
Estée Lauder

Youth Dew was the initial fragrance produced by Estée Lauder and became the first sensational American fragrance hit when it was introduced as bath oil for everyday use. During World War II, perfume had been difficult to obtain, and American women were not accustomed to using fragrance every day. However, they did use bath oils, and Lauder seized upon this, marketing her new fragrance as a bath oil and perfume—a brilliant idea on her part.

Lauder often hinted that Youth Dew was based on a formula her uncle had created for a Russian princess. Whether this story is true or not, women were certainly enthralled by the rich, spicy perfume.

The opulent scent has endured as one of Estée Lauder's most popular fragrances. Youth Dew is a strong, long-lasting scent, perfect for cool weather and dramatic evenings...or anytime you want to be noticed.

Jan's Note: Legend has it that in the 1950s, women often spritzed the back of their French twist hairstyle with Youth Dew to leave a voluptuous trail of perfume as they danced and moved through a room. Or so my mother said...

Scent Type: Spicy Woody Oriental
Top Notes: Orange, bergamot, peach, spices
Heart Notes: Clove, cinnamon, cassie, rose, ylang-ylang, orchid, jasmine
Base Notes: Frankincense, amber, vanilla, oakmoss, clove, musk, patchouli, vetiver, spices

Who's Worn It
Madonna, Duchess of Windsor, Gloria Swanson, Dolores Del Rio, Joan Crawford

Introduced: 1953
***

Zeste Mandarine Pamplemousse
Creed

Creed's Zeste Mandarine Pamplemousse is a rich citrus fragrance suitable for women and men. Bright notes of grapefruit and bergamot are expertly woven with white flowers and lemon bark, but the dominant impression is tangy mandarin, ripe from the orchard. Fresh, cool, invigorating.

Zeste Mandarine Pamplemousse was the first fragrance Olivier Creed created when he became master perfumer for Creed at the age of thirty-two. And it's said that even today, every perfume is still handmade using the infusion method.

The house of Creed dates from 1760 when founder James Henry Creed established his firm in London. In 1854, the firm moved to Paris and continued to flourish under the tutelage of Creed descendants. Today, sixth-generation master perfumer Olivier Creed proudly carries on the family business.

Scent Type: Citrus
Notes: Grapefruit, mandarin, bergamot

Introduced: 1975

Common Ingredients

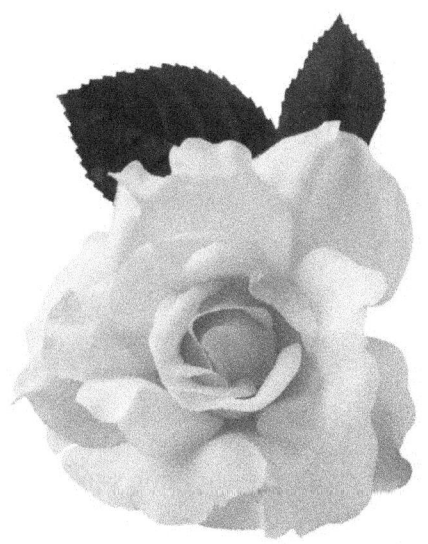

Aldehydes - Organic chemicals derived from natural or synthetic materials. Aldehydes add a vivid, quick quality to top notes. Variations can be powdery, fruity, green, citrusy, floral or woody.

Amber - A fossil resin from the fir tree. Prized for its tenacity, it also adds warm, leathery, powdery elements to a composition. The color amber refers to the color of the resin.

Ambergris - Secretion from the male sperm whale often found floating in the ocean. The Chinese once used it as an aphrodisiac. Ambergris imparts a woody, balsamic odor. Substitutes are used more often today because the natural substance is difficult to obtain.

Ambrette Seed - These plant seeds yield a musky floral, brandy-type aroma.

Anjelica - Oil from the root of the angelica tree which is cultivated in France, Belgium and Germany. It is musky and peppery, with a spicy green quality.

Balsam - Tree resins that exhibit a warm, sweet element. They are generally used as a base fixative.

Basil- A spicy herb with a green impression.

Bay Leaf - A tree leaf valued for its spicy, warm, almost bitter scent.

Bayberry - A shrub with berries from which a waxy substance is taken. Bayberry adds a spicy, woody flair to fragrance.

Benzoin - Balsamic resin from the tropical styrax tree, used as a fixative, imparting a sweet, cocoa-like quality. Benzoin is found in Thailand, Vietnam and Laos.

Bergamot - Oil produced from the peel of the bergamot fruit. The inedible fruit is of the citrus family and is about the size of an orange. The largest bergamot production comes from Calabria, Italy. The fresh, citrus essence is ideal in top notes and eau de cologne.

Black Currant Bud - (see Cassis)

Boronia - Essence taken from the flower of the boronia bush which is mainly found in Australia. Often used in chypre blends, it leaves a spicy-rosy impression.

Broom - This produces a sweet, grassy odor. It is derived from the blossoms of the Mediterranean-area Spanish broom shrub.

Buchu - Substance from the leaves of the buchu herb. It yields a strong minty, camphor odor.

Bulgarian Rose - A highly valued flower in perfumery, grown in Bulgaria's Valley of the Roses at the base of the Balkan mountain range where a Turkish merchant began cultivation centuries ago.

Cardamom - Oil distilled from the cardamom plant, a member of the ginger family. It leaves a spicy floral impression. It is second only to saffron as the world's most expensive spice. In India, cardamom grains are chewed to freshen the breath.

Carnation - This flower gives off a spicy, sensual aroma.

Cassia Oil - Obtained from the leaves of an evergreen tree, valued for its spicy cinnamon-like quality. The oil is also used in cola drinks.

Cassie - Derived from the Acacia farnesiana bush, the cassie absolute produces a spicy floral flavor.

Cassis - Oil taken from the bud of the black currant fruit which is also used in liqueur.

Castoreum - A secretion from the beaver that exudes a leathery quality and is used as a fixative.

Cedarwood - Oil obtained from the juniper cedar tree which is native to Texas. An excellent fixative, it has a distinct wood tone.

Chamomile - A sweet, herbal odor with fruity notes often used to balance floral compositions.

Cinnamon - Oil obtained from the bark and leaves of the *cinnamomum* tree which is native to Southeast Asia and the

Vintage Perfumes

East Indies. It imparts a familiar warm, sweet, spicy odor.

Civet - A glandular secretion from the civet cat used as a fixative. Repugnant by itself, civet blends well and adds a warm, leathery, erotic tone to a composition.

Clary Sage - An herb valued for its sweet, subtle quality.

Clove - Obtained from the clove tree, clove buds are prized for their spicy sweetness. The tree is cultivated in Sri Lanka, Madagascar and Indonesia.

Coriander - Oil from the coriander herb of the parsley family, valued for its spicy aromatic impression.

Costus - Essence from the root of the costus plant of the daisy family, lends warmth to Oriental blends. It has green, violet-like accents.

Coumarin - Obtained from the tonka bean and often created synthetically, produces a sweet, herbal, spicy, hay-like odor, similar to vanilla.

Cyclamen - Essence taken from the heart-shaped flowers of the primrose family.
Eucalyptus - Oil from the leaves of the eucalyptus tree, leaves a strong herbal, camphor impression. Discovered in

Tasmania, it is widely cultivated in Spain, Portugal and Australia and is well priced.

Frangipani - Oil from the sweet, jasmine-like flowers of the frangipani tree.

Frankincense - (see Olibanum)

Galbanum - A gum resin valued for its leafy green, soft balsamic odor. Galbanum is used in many fragrances to provide a pleasing freshness or green lift.

Gardenia - A heady white flower with a strong sweet scent.

Geranium - Oil made from the leaves and stems of the plant. Depending on the variety, it gives off a rosy, minty or fruity essence often used in rosy or spicy compositions.

Ginger - A woody, warm, spicy odor derived from the ginger plant.

Gums - Resins or balsams secreted from plants. Exhibiting a sweet tenacious odor, they are often used as fixatives.

Heliotropin - An aldehyde with a floral almond tone found in pepper oil.

Vintage Perfumes

Honeysuckle - A highly fragrant vine flower but difficult to capture correctly. The essence of honeysuckle is usually re-created by blending a variety of florals.

Hyacinth - A sweet floral that imparts a green impression.

Incense - Made from gums and resins, produces a spicy aroma when burned.

Jasmine - Called the king of flowers, a sweet tiny white flower with a vibrant, smooth aroma. Jasmine is one of the most prized essences in the perfumer's palette. It is grown in France, Morocco, India, Egypt and Spain and must be harvested before sunrise to retain the full amount of its delicate fragrance.

Jonquil - Highly fragrant essence derived from a flower of the narcissus family, rare because it is difficult to distill.

Labdanum - A dark resin obtained from the rockrose herb valued for its leathery odor.

Lavender - From the flowering tops of lavender plants in France, Spain, Morocco and old Yugoslavia, a sweet, light essence with woody floral accents. The oil is used in lavender waters, chypres, fougères and florals. Lavender water is said to have been a favorite of Madame de Pompadour, mistress of Louis XV.

Leather - A smoky, sweet, animal odor crafted from the perfumer's palette. It is warm and persistent.

Lemon - Oil from the lemon rind. It is a zesty, sharp, refreshing essence and is added to brighten many compositions, particularly eau de cologne.

Lilac - Since the essence released by the lilac plant and flower does not accurately portray its aroma, the perfumer re-creates the essence by using jasmine, ylang-ylang, neroli and vanilla.

Lily of the Valley - Also known as muguet, lily of the valley is invented by the perfumer using jasmine, orange blossom, rose, ylang-ylang and chemical additives. The sweet essence is difficult to obtain from the natural flower.

Magnolia - A sweet, highly fragrant flower, also stubborn in releasing its essence. The perfumer re-creates the essence by blending rose, jasmine, neroli and ylang-ylang with aroma chemicals.

Mandarin - Oil from the peel of the mandarin orange fruit, a brisk, sweet essence often used in eau de cologne.

May Rose - Also called rose de mai. The May rose from

Morocco produces a rich, long-lasting oil prized for its full-bodied, diffusive qualities.

Mimosa - A green floral essence obtained from mimosa tree flowers and stems. It imparts a smooth, sweet aroma.

Moss - Earthy essences are derived from a variety of mosses: oakmoss, treemoss, lichen, seaweed and algae.

Muguet (see Lily of the Valley)

Musk - A glandular secretion from the male musk deer of Tibet, China and Nepal, used as a fixative in fine perfumes. It is valued for its woody, animal, erotic impressions, though nowadays it is often created chemically by the perfumer. Soft, sensuous, pervasive.

Narcissus - A highly fragrant yellow and white flower that produces an intense spicy, earthy and sweet straw-like odor. Small amounts are often used to round off floral compositions. Native to Persia, the narcissus flower was carried to China over the silk route in the eighth century.

Neroli - Made from the orange blossoms of the bitter orange tree grown in France, Egypt, Algeria and Morocco. It is light, sweet and spicy and is used in top notes and eau de cologne. It was named for the Duchess of Nerola and was often used to scent gloves.

Nutmeg - Spicy oil derived from the seeds of the South Asian nutmeg tree.

Oakmoss - A lichen grown on oak trees. Its odor is earthy, woody and slightly leathery. It is used as a fixative in many blends, especially chypre.

Olibanum - Also called frankincense. Olibanum is a gum resin from a tree found in Africa and Saudi Arabia. An outstanding fixative, its odor is spicy and balsamic, similar to that of incense.

Opopanax - Derived from a gum resin and similar to myrrh. A woody, sweet fixative.

Orange Blossom - From the white blossoms of the bitter orange tree. It adds a warm, spicy flavor that is often used in floral compositions.

Orange Oil - Produced from the peel of the orange and often used in eau de cologne and floral fragrances. Refreshing, sweet, fruity and crisp.

Orris - One of the most expensive ingredients used in perfumery. It is obtained from the iris plant which is commonly cultivated in Italy. Its odor is violet-like and can be warm, sweet, woody, fruity or floral, depending on the quality.

Osmanthus - Produced from the flowers of the osmanthus tree which is found in Japan, China and Southeast Asia. It has a floral odor with a hint of plum and raisin.

Patchouli - Oil obtained from the leaves of the patchouli plant, a superb fixative. Discovered in India, it is also cultivated in Malaysia and Indonesia. Its odor is earthy, dry, woody and spicy. Patchouli is often used in Oriental and chypre blends.

Petitgrain - Essence derived from the leaves and stems of the bitter orange tree. It has a subtle woody tone similar to neroli. Sweet and floral, petitgrain adds freshness to a fragrance, especially eau de cologne.

Resin - Gum secretions from trees and plants, often used as fixatives.

Rose - Rose oil is also referred to as "otto" or "attar" of rose; these terms refer to perfume oil produced through distillation. There is a wide variety of roses, and the rich oil they produce has the familiar rose aroma, though undertones vary from honey to fruity, spicy to musk, and violet to green.

Called the queen of flowers, it is one of the most precious ingredients in perfumery. Roses bloom just thirty days of the year and must be picked quickly for they lose half their essence by noon. Centifolia and Damascena are popularly cultivated roses. The floral essence is used in rose water, floral, chypre and Oriental compositions. Rose water was said to have been a favorite of Marie Antoinette.

Rose de Mai (see May Rose)

Rosemary - Flowers and leaves of the evergreen rosemary herb of the mint family, distilled for use in perfumery. The oil produces an herbal note that is woody and slightly lavender-like.

Rosewood Oil - Oil obtained from the wood of the rosewood tree, the *aniba rosaeodora* of the laurel family. It gives off a rosy odor, sweet and subtly spicy. Rosewood is often added to eau de cologne.

Sage - A fresh, spicy odor from the sage herb.

Sandalwood - Oil from the sandalwood tree, the evergreen *santalum album* grown in India, Australia and Southeast Asia, though the Indian province of Mysore supplies 85% of all sandalwood. The wood is valued for its aroma and its imperviousness to termites. The trees must mature at least thirty years for the oil to fully develop. An expensive ingredient, sandalwood oil is prized for its fixative quality. Its odor is powdery, balsamic, woody and rich. Sandalwood gives a smooth finish to Oriental, chypre and floral perfumes.

Styrax - A sweet balsam found on the styrax tree, an excellent fixative.

Sweet Pea - A flower oil produced from the fragrant flowering vine, valued for its light, delicate nature.

Tagetes - Essence produced from the tagetes flower which is grown in Spain, Italy and South Africa. The strong essence has an herbal, aromatic personality with fruity undertones.

Thyme - Derived from the flowering herb. Thyme smells sweet and herbaceous--ideal for eau de cologne.

Tonka Bean - Fragrant seeds from native South American trees of the Dipteryx family.

Tuberose - One of the most expensive oils, from a flower known for its rich, sensual aroma. Its cost is due in part to a painstaking processing called enfleurage, an oil extraction method whereby the flowers are pressed into fat, then the oil is separated with alcohol. Tuberose is a perennial plant native to Mexico. The sweet, honey-like aroma adds fullness to many floral fragrances and blends well with gardenia, jonquil and hyacinth.

Vanilla - Made from the fruit and seeds of a climbing orchid vine. It has pods, or capsules, encasing the beans. Vanilla is an impressive sweet fixative used in many Oriental, amber and floral perfumes.

Vanillin - Can be produced naturally from the vanilla pod, as well as certain balsams and benzoins. It can also be made synthetically. Its sweet, strong odor is similar to vanilla, but lacks the depth of vanilla. Vanillin blends well with vanilla to produce a round, full-bodied vanilla aroma.

Vetiver - A grass grown in Haiti, Réunion Island, Brazil, China and Southeast Asia. It has a woody, earthy quality enhanced by a moist balsamic accent. A superb fixative, vetiver is an important component in chypre blends.

Violet - The violet flower yields such a minute amount of oil that it is cost prohibitive to extract. Instead, the violet aroma is created chemically for use in perfumery.

Violet Leaf - Oil from the leaves of the violet plant, valued for its cucumbery green and peppery herbal aroma, with touches of violet and iris. Parma, Italy is known for its violet production.

Vintage Perfumes

Ylang-Ylang - From Tagalog for "flower of flowers." This oil comes from the flower of ylang-ylang trees grown in Madagascar, Indonesia, Comoros and the Philippines. The rich oil has a jasmine-like aroma and sweet balsamic accents. Used in many floral and Oriental compositions, ylang-ylang smooths and rounds bitter notes, adding warmth and grace.

JAN MORAN

Bibliography and Sources

"The Effect of Fragrance on the Mood of a Woman at Midlife," "Mood Benefits of Fragrance." *Aroma-Chology Review,* Vol. II, No. 1.

Beauty Fashion. Various editions.

Booth, Nancy. *Perfumes, Splashes & Colognes.* Pownal, Vermont: Storey Communications, 1997.

Booth, Nancy. *Scentsations.* Buckingham Impressions, 1998.

Bork, Karl-Heinz; Elke Doerrier; Arturetto Landi; Egon Oelkers; Peter Woerner; Lothar Kuemper. *Fragrance Guide: Feminine Notes, Masculine Notes.* Hamburg, Germany: Glöss Verlag, 1991.

Science & Technology. "No One's Sniffing at Aroma Research Now." *Business Week,* December 23, 1991, 82.

Chanel, Inc. *Chanel Fragrances.* New York: Chanel, Inc., 1991.

"How to Buy a Fragrance." *Consumer Reports*, December 1993, 765-773.

"All Passion Scent." *Country Living*.

"The Raison d'être of the Fragrance Foundation: Past, Present and Future." *Dragoco Report*, January 1991, 3-9.

Etherington-Smith, Meredith. *Patou*. New York: St. Martin's, 1983.

Fischer-Rizzi, Susanne. *Complete Aromatherapy Handbook: Essential Oils for Radiant Health*. New York: Sterling Publishing, 1990.

The Fragrance Foundation. *The Facts and Fun of Fragrance*. New York: Fragrance Foundation, 1992.

The Fragrance Foundation. *The Fragrance Foundation Reference Guide 1999*. New York: Fragrance Foundation, 1999.

The Fragrance Foundation. *Fragrance and Olfactory Directory*. New York: Fragrance Foundation, 1981.

The Fragrance Foundation. *The History, the Mystery, the Enjoyment of Fragrance*. New York: Fragrance Foundation.

Gaborit, Jean-Yves. *Perfumes: The Essences and Their Bottles*. New York: Rizzoli, 1985.

Happi. June 1994 through January 2015.

Israel, Lee. *Estée Lauder: Beyond the Magic*. New York: MacMillan Publishing Co., 1985.

Vintage Perfumes

Kaufman, William. *Perfume*. New York: E.P. Dutton & Co., 1974.

"History of an Ancient Art," "Lalique Parfums," "Recipe for a Fragrance." *Lalique Magazine*, Winter 1993, 4-11.

Lauder, Estée. *Estée: A Success Story*. New York: Random House, 1985.

Lawless, Julia. *The Encyclopedia of Essential Oils*. New York: Barnes & Noble Books, 1995.

"Scientists Say Aromas Have Major Effect on Emotions." *Los Angeles Times*, May 31, 1991, B3.

Monroe, Valerie. "How to Smell Really Wonderful." *McCall's*, September 1993, 140, 182.

"Scent System." *Mirabella*, October 1991, 142-143.

Morris, Edwin T. *Fragrance: The Story of Perfume from Cleopatra to Chanel*. New York: Charles Scribner's Sons, 1984.

Müller, Julia. *The H&R Book of Perfume*. Hamburg, Germany: Glöss Verlag, 1992

"The Intimate Sense." *National Geographic*, September 1986, 324-360.

"Discovery May Unlock Secret of Smell." *New York Times*, April 5, 1991, A1.

Newman, Cathy. *Perfume: The Art and Science of Scent*. National Geographic Society, 1998.

Ohrbach, Barbara Milo. *A Bouquet of Flowers: Sweet Thoughts, Recipes, and Gifts from the Garden with "The Language of Flowers."* New York: Clarkson N. Potter, Inc., 1990.

Olfactory Research Fund Ltd. *Living Well With Your Sense of Smell.* New York: Olfactory Research Fund Ltd., 1992.

Pavia, Fabienne. *The World of Perfume.* New York: Knickerbocker Press, 1996.

"Dollars and Scents." *Philadelphia Inquirer*, September 29, 1991, section J.

Pickles, Sheila. *The Language of Flowers.* New York: Harmony Books, 1989.

Scents & Style. November 1995 through December 1998.

"The Coming Age of Aroma-Chology." *Soap/Cosmetics/Chemical Specialties*, April 1991, 30-32.

Von Furstenberg, Diane. *Diane von Fürstenberg's Book of Beauty.* New York: Simon & Schuster, 1976.

Lab Notes. "Sniffing Heliotrope Helps MRI Patients Sit Still." *Wall Street Journal*, August 8, 1991.

"What the Nose Knows." *Washington Post*, July 26, 1992.

Women's Wear Daily. Various editions.

Green, Annette; Fragrance Foundation. Interviewed by author. October 1993.

Vintage Perfumes

Hayman, Gale; Gale Hayman Beverly Hills. Interviewed by author. October 1993.

Mosbacher, Georgette, and Paulsin, Lyn; Exclusives. Interviewed by author. October 1993

Completed questionnaires, interviews, information, permissions, media kits and photography were supplied, in part or in total, by the following companies:

Adipar, Antonia's Flowers, Laura Ashley, Barclay Perfumes, Brandselite, Benetton Cosmetics, Bijan, Boucheron, Bulgari, Cassini Parfums, Caesars World Merchandising, Chanel, Liz Claiborne, Compar, Cosmair, Dionne Inc., Christian Dior, Erox, Escada, EuroCos, Marilyn Evins, Exclusives, Alice Fixx, The Fragrance Foundation, French Fragrances, Givenchy, Annick Goutal, Guerlain, Fred Hayman, Gale Hayman, Hermès Parfums, Jivago, Donna Karan Beauty Company, Key West Aloe, La Merveille Cie, Lancaster Group, Ralph Lauren Fragrances, L'Oréal, Parfums Lucien Lelong, Marina Maher, Marilyn Miglin, Jessica McClintock, Madeleine Mono, Georgette Mosbacher, Neiman Marcus, Niro, Nordstrom's, Olfactory Research Fund, William Owen, Parfums International, Parlux, Jean Patou, Perfumania, Prescriptives, Revlon, Riviera Concepts, Rochas, Chen Sam, Paul Sebastian, Tiffany, Ungaro, Vepro, Diane Von Furstenberg, XEL, and others.

JAN MORAN

Vintage Perfumes Book Club Discussion

After reading *Vintage Perfumes*, share your thoughts on perfumery with your book club. These perfume-related discussion questions can ignite lively discussions and powerful memories for club members.

1. What are your favorite classic perfumes? Do you have any cherished memories of when you wore these fragrances?

2. Many people recall the perfume their mother or father, grandparent, or another favorite person wore. Do you have any vintage fragrance memories of family members or other loved ones?

3. What we think of as classic designer perfumes today were envisioned and brought to life by highly creative entrepreneurs who often had fascinating life stories. Would you like to share the history or memories of vintage fashion designers such as Coco Chanel, Christian Dior, or Jean Patou?

4. In the medical field, scents are sometimes used to help patients retrieve long forgotten memories. Have you ever experienced a sudden memory return when you detected a certain aroma? Do particular scents bring back memories for you?

5. Has reading *Vintage Perfumes* helped you understand the fragrance categories and why you are drawn toward certain notes or perfume families? Why do you think this is? Which ones are your favorites?

6. Do you ever use the wardrobe approach to selecting perfumes? For example, do you have a favorite perfume for summer? How about for black-ties affairs or date night?

7. The olfactory sense is the most overlooked sense in writing, but it's a powerfully evocative one. When you read fiction, do you find yourself more immersed in a scene when the author employs the sense of smell? Do you notice it?

8. Can you think of any examples where an author used scent or perfume to create a setting, conjure a memory, or draw a character?

9. Do you have any perfume traditions you'd like to share?

Excerpt from *Scent of Triumph* Novel

Read on for an excerpt from *Scent of Triumph*, Jan Moran's historical novel about a courageous French perfumer during World War II (published by St. Martin's Press).

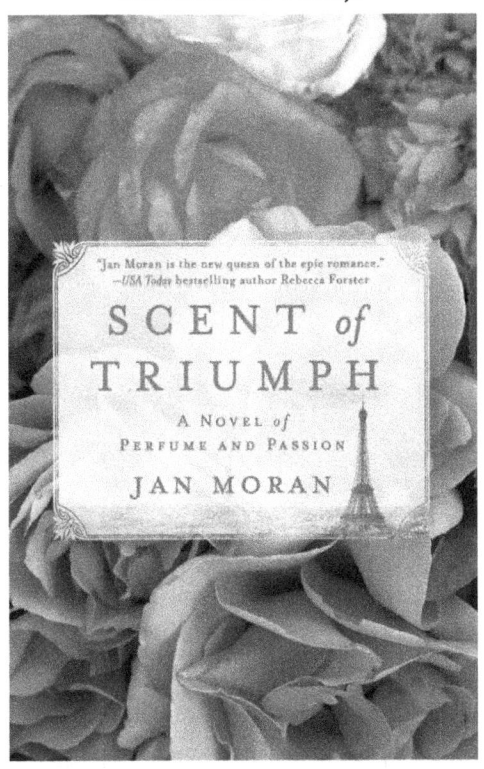

JAN MORAN

Vintage Perfumes

Chapter One

A rose, the symbol of love, the queen of the perfumer's palette. How then, does the perfume of war intoxicate even the most reasonable of men?
– From the perfume journal of Danielle Bretancourt

3 September, 1939
Atlantic Ocean

Danielle Bretancourt von Hoffman braced herself against the mahogany-paneled stateroom wall, striving for balance as she flung open a brass porthole, seeking a moment of respite she knew would never be. A damp, kelp-scented wind—a harbinger of the storm ahead—whistled through the cabin, assaulting her nose with its raw intensity, but the sting of salty spray did little to assuage the fear she had for her little boy.

Nicky was only six years old. *Why, oh why did I agree to leave him behind?* She had wanted to bring him, but her husband had disagreed, saying he was far too young for such an arduous journey. As a trained scientist, his arguments were always so logical, so sensible. Against her instinct, she had given in to Max. It was settled; in their absence her mother-in-law, Sofia, would care for Nicky on their old family estate in Poland.

Danielle kept her eyes focused on the horizon as the *Newell-Grey Explorer* slanted upward, slicing through the peak of a cresting wave. The ocean liner creaked and pitched as it heaved through the turbulent gray waters of the Atlantic on its voyage from New York to England. Silently, Danielle urged it onward, anxious to return home.

Her usually sturdy stomach churned in rhythm with the sea. Was it morning sickness, anxiety, or the ravaging motion of the sea? Probably all three, she decided. Just last week she'd been so wretchedly ill that she'd seen a doctor, who confirmed her pregnancy. The timing couldn't be worse.

She blinked against the stiff breeze, her mind reeling. When they'd heard reports of the new agreement between Germany and Russia, they'd cut their business short to hurry home. Had it been just two days since they'd learned the devastating news that Nazi forces had invaded Poland?

Someone knocked sharply on the door. Gingerly crossing the room, Danielle opened the door to Jonathan Newell-Grey, heir apparent to the British shipping line that bore his family name. His tie hung from his collar and his sleeves were rolled up, exposing muscular forearms taut from years of sailing. A rumpled wool jacket hung over one shoulder.

Vintage Perfumes

Danielle and Max had met Jon on their outbound voyage to New York several weeks ago. They had become good friends, dining together regularly on the ship, and later in the city. Well-traveled and physically fit, Jon loved to explore and dine on fine food, and insisted on taking them to the best restaurants in New York, as well as little-known nooks that served authentic French and German fare, assuring Max and Danielle of a salve for their homesickness after their relocation. During their time in New York, Max worked tirelessly, tending to details for their pending cross-Atlantic move, so they both appreciated having a knowledgeable friend to call on for help.

With his gregarious yet gracious manner, Jon had helped them find a good neighborhood for their family, introduced them to his banker, and even explained some of the odd American colloquialisms they couldn't understand, as they all laughed together over well-aged bottles of his favorite Bordeaux. They had all climbed the Empire State Building together, and one night they saw a play on Broadway, and even danced to Benny Goodman's big band into the late evening hours. Jon also went to the World's Fair with them, where their crystal perfume bottles were featured in a potential business partner's display. Danielle and Max were both glad they'd met Jon, a man who embraced life with spirit and joie de vivre, and they looked forward to their new life in America far from the threat of Hitler's forces.

But now, with news of the invasion, Max and Danielle's

guarded optimism for their future had turned to distress over their family's safety.

"*Bonjour*," she said, glad to see Jon. "Any news yet?"

"None." He pushed a hand through his unruly chestnut hair, droplets of water spray glistening on his tanned face. "The captain has called a meeting at fifteen hundred hours for all passengers traveling on Polish and German passports."

"But I still hold a French passport."

"You'll need to attend, Danielle." His hoarse voice held the wind of the sea. "Of course, but—" As another sharp pitch jerked through the ship, Jon caught her by the shoulders and kept her from falling. He moved intuitively with the ship's motion, a testament to his years at sea.

"Steady now, lass," Jon said, a small smile playing on his lips. He stared past her out the porthole, his dark eyes riveted on the ocean's whitecapped expanse. Blackened, heavily laden clouds crossed the sun, casting angled shadows across his face.

Embarrassed, Danielle touched the wall for support. She recalled the strange sense of foreboding she'd had upon waking. She was blessed—or cursed—with an unusually keen prescience. Frowning, she asked, "Can the ship withstand this storm?"

"Sure, she's a fine, seaworthy vessel, one of the finest in the world. This weather's no match for her." He turned back to her, his jaw set. His usual jovial nature had turned solemn. "Might even be rougher seas ahead, but we'll make England

Vintage Perfumes

by morning."

Danielle nodded, but still, *she knew*. Anxiety coursed through her; something seemed terribly wrong. Her intuition came in quiet flashes of pure knowledge. She couldn't force it, couldn't direct it, and knew better than to discuss it with anyone, especially her husband. She was only twenty-six; Max was older, wiser, and told her that her insights were rubbish. Max wasn't really insulting her; he had studied science at the university in Germany, and he simply didn't believe anything that couldn't be scientifically proven.

Jon touched her arm in a small, sympathetic movement. "Anything I can do to help?"

"Not unless you perform miracles." Jon's rough fingers were warm against her skin, and an ill-timed memory from a few days ago shot through her mind. Danielle loved to dance, and with Max's encouragement, she and Jon had shared a dance while Max spoke to the captain at length after dinner. Danielle remembered Jon's soft breath, his musky skin, his hair curling just above his collar. He'd been interested in all she had to say, from her little boy to her work at Parfums Bretancourt, her family's perfumery in the south of France. But when she'd rested her head against his chest, it was his skin, his natural scent, which was utterly unique and intriguingly virile, that mesmerized her.

A third-generation perfumer, Danielle had an acute sense of smell. Her olfactory skills were paramount in the laboratory, but at times this acuity proved socially awkward.

Jon's scent still tingled in her nose, taunting her dreams, its musky animal appeal relentless in the recesses of her mind. His memory crept into her mind more than she knew it should. *After all,* she told herself firmly, *I am a happily married woman.*

Danielle forced the scene from her mind, took a step back out of modesty. She caught sight of herself in the mirror, her thick auburn hair in disarray, her lip rouge smeared. She smoothed her celadon green silk day dress—one of her own designs her dressmaker had made—and drew her fingers across her pale skin. "I've been apprehensive about this trip from the beginning."

"Have you heard anything else from your mother-in-law?"

"Not since we spoke in New York. And my mother's last cable said they haven't arrived." When she and Max had heard the news, they called Max's mother, Sofia, and told her to leave immediately with Nicky for Paris, where Danielle's parents had a spacious apartment in the sixteenth arrondissement, a fine neighborhood in the heart of Paris. Sofia's voice had sounded dreadful; they hadn't realized she was so sick. *What if she isn't well enough to travel?* Wincing with remorse, Danielle fought the panic that rose in her throat, fearful for her mother-in-law.

"They have to get out of Poland." Jon touched her cheek.

Reflexively, she turned into the comfort of his hand,

inhaling, her heart aching, his scent—at once both calming and unsettling—edged with the smell of the sea and a spiced wood blend she normally could have recognized in an instant. But now, Nicky was ever present in her mind. Danielle pressed her eyes closed and stifled a sob.

"Max is resourceful," Jon said, trailing his hand along her face. "He'll manage."

But can he? she wondered. Max had planned everything, from organizing their move to New York, to returning to Poland to close their home. He'd arranged their immigration to the United States, and he was also trying to bring their most valued employees with them for the business. *He'd made everything sound so sensible.*

Max was German, born in Berlin to an aristocratic family. When Max was young, his mother had inherited her family's estate and crystal and glass factory in Poland. Sofia and her husband, Karl, along with Karl's orphaned nephew, Heinrich, moved into the castle, which had originally been built as a wedding gift in 1820 for Sofia's ancestors. While the men set about rebuilding the factory and the business, Sofia tended to the home, a masterpiece of romantic English neo-Gothic style. After Max and Danielle married, Danielle had thrown her considerable energy into helping Sofia restore the grand salons and chambers, the arboretum, the gardens and ponds. And yet, Danielle missed her craft, retreating whenever she could to the perfumery organ—a curved workbench with rows that held essential oils and other perfumery materials—she had installed in their quarters, to conjure her aromatic artistry in solitude. Perfumery fed her soul; her urge to create could not be repressed.

The ship pitched again, sending the porthole door banging against the paneled wall. Shifting easily with the vessel's sharp motions, Jon caught it, secured the latch.

He moved toward her, and she could almost sense the adrenaline surging through his muscular frame. Leaning closer, he lifted a strand of hair limp with sea mist from her forehead. "If I don't see Max, you'll tell him about the captain's meeting?"

"We'll be there." She caught another whiff of his sea air–tinged skin, and this time a vivid sensory image flashed across her mind. A leather accord, patchouli, a heart of rose melding with the natural scent of his skin, warm, intriguing...then she recognized it—Spanish Leather. *An English composition. Trumper.* But the way he wore it was incredible; the *parfum* blended with his own natural aroma in such a fascinating manner. She was drawn in, aching to be swept farther into his scent, but she quickly retreated half a step. *This is not the time.*

His expression softened and he let her hair fall from his fingers as he studied her, his dark-browed, hazel-flecked eyes taking in every feature of her face.

Danielle stepped back, and Jon's gaze trailed back to the sea, his eyes narrowed against the sun's thinning rays, scanning the surface.

Vintage Perfumes

She matched his dark gaze. "Something unusual out there?"

"Might be German U-boats. *Unterseeboots.* The most treacherous of submarines. Bloody hell, they are. But don't worry, Danielle, the Newell-Greys always look after their passengers." He left, closing the door behind him.

U-boats? So it was possible. She touched a trembling finger to her lips. But that wasn't the only thought that made her uncomfortable. Jon's friendly, casual way with her increasingly struck a chord within her. Fortunately, Max was too much the aristocrat to make a fuss over nothing. *And it is nothing,* she thought. She loved her husband. *But that scent...*her mind whirred. *Fresh, spicy, woodsy...I can recreate sea freshness, blend it with patchouli....*

Abruptly, the ship lurched. Cutlery clattered across a rimmed burl wood table, her books tumbled against a wall. She braced herself through the crashing swell, one hand on the doorjamb, another shielding her womb. There were so many urgent matters at hand. *Our son, our family, our home.* She pulled her mind back to the present.

When the ship leveled, she spied on the floor a navy blue cap she'd knitted for Nicky. He'd dropped it at the train station, and she'd forgotten to give it to Sofia. She cradled it in her hand and stroked it, missing him and the sound of his voice, then pressed the cap to her nose, drinking in his little boy smell that still clung to the woolen fibers. Redolent of milk and grass and straw and chocolates, it also called to mind sweet perspiration droplets glistening on his flushed cheeks. They often played tag in the estate's lush, sprawling gardens, laughing and frolicking, feeding the migratory ducks that visited their ponds, or strolling beneath the protective leafy boughs of ancient, towering trees. She brushed away tears that spilled onto her cheeks.

She picked up her purse to put his cap inside, and then paused to look at the photograph of Nicky she carried. His eyes crinkled with laughter, he'd posed with his favorite stuffed toy, a red-striped monkey with black button eyes she'd sewn for him. Nicky was an adorable bundle of blond-headed energy. A streak of fear sliced through her. She stuffed the cap into her purse and snapped it shut.

The door opened and Max strode into the stateroom, his proud face ashen, his lean, angular body rigid with what Danielle knew was stress.

"Jon just left," she said. "There's a meeting—"

"I know, he is behind me," Max said, clipping the words in his formal, German-accented English. He smacked his onyx pipe against his hand, releasing the sweet smoky scent of his favorite vanilla tobacco.

Jon appeared at the door. "Shall we go?"

The muscles in Max's jaw tightened. He slipped his pipe into the pocket of his tailored wool jacket. "I need a drink first. You, Jon?"

"Not now, mate."

Max moved past Danielle to the liquor cabinet,

staggering slightly as the ship pitched. He brushed against her vanity and sent her red leather traveling case crashing to the floor.

Danielle gasped. Bottles smashed against one another inside as the case tumbled. The lid burst open, and scents of jasmine, rose, orange blossom, bergamot, berries, vanilla, cedar, and sandalwood exploded like brilliant fireworks.

"Oh, Max, my perfumes." She gathered the hem of her silk dress and sank to her knees, heartsick. These were all the perfumes she had with her; she could hardly remember a day when she hadn't worn one of her *parfum* creations. She knew Max hadn't meant to destroy her precious potions, but now there was nothing she could do but gather the pieces. With two fingers, she fished a crystal shard and a carnelian cap from the jagged mess. "Max, would you hand me the wastebasket?"

"I, I didn't mean to…" Looking worried, Max turned away and reached for the vodka, sighing in resignation. "Just leave it, Danielle. The cabin boy will see to it."

Jon knelt beside her. "Did you make all these?"

"Yes, I did. And the case was Max's wedding gift to me."

"These are beautiful works of art, Danielle. Max told me you were once regarded as the child prodigy of perfumery." He took a sharp piece from her. "Don't hurt yourself, I'll send someone to clean this up while you're gone."

She caught his eye and mouthed a silent thank-you, then rose and opened the porthole. A gust caught her long hair and slapped it across her face, stinging her flushed cheeks.

Staring at the ocean, a quiet intuitive knowledge crept into her consciousness. *It's true*, she thought, and spun around. "Jon said there might be U-boats out there."

She watched Max pour a shot, then pause with his glass in midair, his intellectual mind whirring, weighing the probabilities. She knew her husband well; she saw his eyes flash with a moment of intensity, then clear into twin pools of lucid blue as he decided the odds were against it. "Impossible," he said.

"Anything is possible." Jon brushed broken crystal into the wastebasket and straightened.

Danielle thoughts reeled back over the morning. "Is that why we've been zigzagging?"

Jon shot a look at Max. "Smart one, your wife. Not just an artist, I see." One side of his mouth tugged to a reassuring grin, shifting the deep cleft in his chin. "I'll grant you that, Danielle, but it's just a safety measure. U-boats aren't a threat to passenger liners."

Pressure built in her head. "Like the *Lusitania*?"

"A disaster like that couldn't happen today," Jon said, rubbing the indentation in his chin. "Every captain checks Lloyd's Register. It's clear that we're a passenger ship. Even so, there are rules of war; an initial shot across the bow must be fired in warning. And England is not at war."

"Not yet." Max tossed the vodka down his throat and gave a wry, thin-lipped grin. "So is that why you have been holding court in the stern, Jon?"

Vintage Perfumes

"I confess, you're on to me, old boy. But seriously, we'd have time to signal to a vessel that we're not armed. Even a submarine must abide by these rules of war. Even the Nazis."

Nazis. The word filled Danielle with dread. What the Nazis were doing to Jews in Germany was unconscionable. New laws required that yellow stars for identification be sewn onto clothing. *Imagine.* Jewish businesses were being destroyed, entire families beaten or killed. These were *German* citizens, many of whom had lived in Germany for generations. It didn't matter how educated they were, whether they were young or old, wealthy or poor. A chill crept along her spine. "We've taken too long, Max. We have to get Nicky and your mother out now."

"The Polish army is not yet defeated, my dear," Max said quietly, pouring another shot. "Try to have patience."

"How can you be so calm?" Her voice hitched in despair. Her father was from an old French family, long recognized in French society. Danielle's mother was Jewish, so by German law Nicky was one-quarter Jewish. "You know what could happen to Nicky."

"We've been over this. Nicky is just a child." Max looked weary, the prominent veins in his high forehead throbbing as he spoke. "You were raised in your father's faith, you are Catholic. Nicky was also baptized. How would the Nazis find out anything different?"

But she knew they had ways. She pressed her hand to her mouth, consumed with worry and guilt. *Why did I agree to leave Nicky?*

Max gulped his drink, and then glanced at Jon. "We should go now." Max walked to the door. Without turning he paused, his voice thick. "I am sorry for your perfumes, Danielle. I am sorry for everything."

Danielle sucked in her breath. Max only drank when he was frustrated, when he had no clear answers. *And he seldom offers an apology.* To him, it was a sign of defeat, a sign that his scientific mind, or measured actions, had betrayed him. Max took pride in providing financially for his family, their well-being was his constant concern, especially that of Nicky, his beloved son. Danielle was the heart of their marriage, and she always felt safe with him. *Except today,* she thought, fear gripping her body like a vine. *Today is different.*

Jon opened the door, held it for them. She snatched her purse and followed Max.

Passengers jostled past in the crowded corridor and Danielle could feel anxiety rising in the air like a heat wave, smell the sour perspiration—like coddled milk left in the sun—emanating from panicked, angry passengers. Ordinary perspiration smelled different when tainted with fear. "Rotten Krauts," they heard people say. She saw Max stiffen against the verbal assaults.

When they came to the open-air promenade deck, Danielle glanced out over the sea, but she could see little in the gathering mist.

Jon followed her gaze. "We've got a heavy fog rolling in."

Vintage Perfumes

The air held the ozone-scented promise of rain. "It's so dim," she said. "Jon, why aren't the running lights on?"

"We're blacked out for security."

There's more to it, she thought, her neck tightening with trepidation.

They arrived at the first-class lounge, where tense passengers crowded shoulder to shoulder. Jon excused himself to take his place near the front as the owner representative. A hush spread when the grim-faced captain approached the podium.

"Thank you for your attention," the captain began. "Two days ago, Hitler's Nazi Germany violated a European peace agreement. Now, on the wireless we have a reply from the Prime Minister of the United Kingdom."

He nodded to a crew member. The loudspeakers crackled to life and a nervous murmur rippled across the room.

England was on the airwaves.

The radio announcer was speaking about Poland. "*Blitzkrieg*," he called the German attack on the country.

"Lightning war," Max translated, shaking his head. He flexed his jaw, and Danielle could see veins bulging from his temples as he sought to control unfamiliar emotions.

"Oh, no." Danielle turned her face against Max's chest, the tentacles of terror slithering into her brain. *It has begun,* she thought, *and so horribly.* She trembled. *My poor Nicky, dear Sofia. Mon Dieu, what's happening to them? How* frightened they must be.

Max slid a finger under her chin and lifted her face to his, wiping tears from her eyes with an awkward gesture. "It's my fault, I should have already relocated our family. I didn't realize this would happen so quickly."

The tortured guilt in his expression tore at her soul. *He has failed. All his plans, all his actions, were to protect our family.* She averted her eyes from his pain, trying to calm her breathing as people wailed around her.

The radio crackled again. "*And now, Prime Minister Chamberlain.*"

"*This morning the British ambassador in Berlin handed the German government a final note stating that, unless we heard from them by eleven o'clock that they were prepared at once to withdraw their troops from Poland, a state of war would exist between us.*"

Chamberlain's voice sounded burdened, yet resolute. "*I have to tell you now that no such undertaking has been received, and that consequently, this country is at war with Germany.*"

A collective gasp filled the room, and Danielle sank against Max for support. He wrapped his arms around her, murmuring in her ear. "We'll find them, they'll soon be safe." *But is he reassuring me or himself?*

At the end of the broadcast, the captain stepped aside and Jon strode to the podium. Jon's baritone voice boomed over the murmuring tide. "Tomorrow, when we arrive,

Vintage Perfumes

Newell-Grey agents will be available to assist and accommodate you. We shall keep you informed as we receive additional information."

Danielle pressed a hand to her mouth. *Who knew it would come to this?* A sudden clamminess overtook her, and her nausea returned with unbridled force. Tearing herself from Max, she bolted through the crowd, bumping against other passengers as she raced to the outer deck. She reached the railing, leaned over, gulped for air. Her stomach convulsed in a dry heave as the wind whipped the celadon scarf from her neck.

"Danielle," Max called, following her. Jon rushed after them.

I can't stand this, she thought, anguish ripping through her as images of Nicky and Sofia filled her mind. Max and Jon reached her side, and the three of them stood gazing through the shifting fog into the bleak waters below as Danielle clung to the railing, one arm clutching her abdomen, pressing her fevered cheek against the cold metal railing for relief

Max draped an arm across her shoulders, rubbing her back, and looked across at Jon. "Her morning sickness is much worse with this pregnancy."

But Jon's eyes were fixed on the ocean. His face froze.

A sleek, narrow wake rippled the broken surface.

"What the—" began Max.

"Good God, get down," Jon bellowed. He leapt across

Max and Danielle, his powerful body crashing them to the deck.

Danielle hit the wooden boards with such force that her shoulder cracked and her eyes blurred. *My baby*, she thought frantically, curling instinctively around her midsection, wrapping her arms around her torso and drawing up her knees to shield her unborn child.

In the next instant, a violent impact shot them across the deck. An explosion ripped into the bowels of the great ship. Screams pierced the haze, and the ship's massive framework buckled with a roar.

"Torpedoes," Jon shouted. He crushed his hand over Danielle's head and cursed under his breath. "Stay down."

An icy burst enveloped them like a sheet and soaked them to the flesh. Danielle gasped in terror. *Mon Dieu!* She could hear Max scrambling behind her, sliding on the slippery deck. *Protect us*, she prayed, keeping her head down and pressing her chin against her chest.

Another explosion rocked the ship. Wood and metal twisted with a grating screech as the ship listed to the starboard side, rolling like a wounded whale. The ship groaned and folded under her own weight, frigid salt water pouring into her open wounds.

Jon struggled to his feet. "Take my hand, Danielle, we must reach the lifeboats. This way, Max." Jon dragged Danielle behind him. "Nazi bastards." He stopped, and pulled his shoulders back. He turned to face the dazed crowd behind him.

"Attention." Jon's voice rang with urgent authority. "We must proceed quickly and calmly to the lifeboats."

Amid the chaos, people turned to follow.

Danielle reached for Jon's hand again, stumbling on something in her haste. She wiped stinging water from her eyes and blinked. A woman she'd met yesterday lay bloodied at her feet. She smothered a scream, and then reached down to help the woman.

Jon caught her arm. "Don't, it's no use. She's gone."

"No, she can't be," Danielle cried. She'd never seen a dead person before. Except for the blood soaking the deck beneath her, the woman appeared merely unconscious. *This can't be happening.* Then she saw that the back of the woman's skull was gone and she started to retch.

Jon shoved his handkerchief into her hand to wipe her mouth. "Keep going," he yelled.

Soon they came upon a lifeboat that dangled above them like a toy.

"Max, give us a hand, we haven't much time. Danielle, wrap your arms around the rail." Jon slicked his wet hair back from his eyes and grabbed a line. Max fought for balance, staggering to the lifeboat.

Water poured over the rail and mixed with the dead woman's blood, sloshing across the deck and staining it a deep crimson. All around them people slid across the tilting deck, screaming in hysteria. Danielle lost her balance, along with one leather pump that tumbled into the pandemonium. She kicked off her other shoe and clung to the railing.

Jon and Max began to toss life vests from the boat into the crowd.

Danielle's heart raced at the sight of the life vests. "Are we...are we going to sink?"

Jon's jaw twitched. "Just put on one of these."

"But I can't swim," she cried, her voice rising with fright.

"You won't have to if you're wearing this."

Despite her panic, Danielle fumbled with the strings on the vest. Jon and Max worked feverishly to free the lifeboats. Within moments, several crew members arrived and began to herd women and children into the boats.

Max checked her vest, tugged her knots to strengthen them, and kissed Danielle while the first boat was lowered. "Go now, I'll see you soon."

She peered at the lifeboat and terror gripped her chest. *No, not this.* She'd never liked small crafts, had nearly drowned off one when she was a child. Danielle stood rooted in horror at the thought of climbing into a boat.

Jon waved his arm at her. "Get in," he roared, his voice gravelly.

She turned to Max, her eyes pleading with him. "Max, I can't."

"Yes, you can. I'll be right behind you, my love." Despite the bulky life vest, Max pressed her to him and kissed her again, reassuring her.

Vintage Perfumes

Jon grabbed her arm with such force that Danielle yelped with pain. "Danielle, people are waiting."

"No, Jon, I–I can't get into that boat. I'll stay with Max."

"Bloody hell, you will." Jon's eyes flamed with urgency, startling her. "For God's sake, woman, get your wits about you. What happened to your famous French courage?"

Max threw Jon a wary glance, and then nodded to her. "He's right, you must go now."

Indignant, Danielle jerked her arm from Jon. "I'll show you courage." She stepped into the boat, barefoot, still clutching her purse.

As she settled unsteadily into the boat, a man with a sobbing young child rushed toward them. "Please, will someone take my boy?"

Danielle thought of her own little boy, shot a glare at Jon. "I will." She reached for the frightened child.

"His name is Joshua. You will take care of my boy?"

"I give you my word." She prayed someone would do the same for her Nicky, if need be. She hugged the tearful child, sweet with a milky smell, to her breast. Joshua was the same size as Nicky and it was all she could do to keep from calling his name.

Jon gave the signal and the lifeboat plunged into the choppy ocean. Danielle squeezed her eyes shut and bent over the boy to protect him as a wave hurtled toward the boat and broke against the wooden bow, blasting them with an icy shock and plastering their hair and clothes to their skin.

Her teeth chattering, Danielle looked back at the great ship. She was taking on water fast. All around them lifeboats crashed into the sea amid the most heart-wrenching cries she'd ever heard.

She strained to see through the fog and the frantic crowd, but couldn't spot Max or Jon. The *Newell-Grey Explorer*, the fine ship that bore Jon's family name, was giving way, slipping to her death. For a moment, the ship heaved against the crushing weight of her watery grave.

Danielle's eyes were glued to the horrific scene. Then, she remembered something she'd once heard. *We've got to act.* Alarmed, she turned to the young crew member with them. "When a ship goes down, the force can suck others down with it. We've got to get out of here."

Dazed with shock, he made no reply.

Frustrated, she turned to the elderly woman next to her. "Here, take little Joshua, hold him tightly." She gave the woman her purse, too.

Another woman let out a cry. "But what will we do?"

"We've got to row," Danielle shouted. "Who'll help me?" She had watched her brother Jean-Claude row often enough. *Surely I can manage this,* she thought desperately.

A stout Irishwoman with coppery red hair spoke up. "I might be third class, but I'm a first-class rower."

"Good." Danielle's resolve hardened and she moved into position. She tucked her soggy silk dress between her legs, its dye trailing green across the white deck, and grabbed an oar.

"Together, now stroke, and—no, wait." When she lifted her arms to row, the life vest bunched up around her neck, inhibiting her movement. She glanced at little Joshua and realized he had no life vest. She tore the vest strings open, shrugged out of it, and gave it to the elderly woman. "Put it on him."

"All right, now stroke," the Irishwoman called. "Steady, and stroke, and stroke."

Danielle pulled hard against the oars, struggling for rhythm, though splinters dug into her hands and her thin sleeves ripped from the strain.

They were some distance out when she looked up. The immense ship, the jewel of the fleet, gave one last, mournful wail as she conceded defeat. The ship disappeared into the Atlantic blackness, leaving only a burgeoning swell of water and a spiral of smoke in her wake.

Where's Max? And Jon? Did they make it off the ship? She couldn't watch anymore, she turned her back to the ship, numb to the cold.

And there, in the distance, she saw it. A strange vessel was breaking the surface. As it crested, she saw on its side in block print the letter *U* and a series of numbers. *A U-boat.* Treacherous, Jon had said. *And deadly.*

Danielle narrowed her eyes. *So, this is the enemy, this is who holds Poland—and my family—captive.*

A scorching rage exploded within her and sent her to the boat's edge, her hands fisted white, shaking with fury. *Look* at them, surveying their handiwork, the bastards. Steadying herself on the bow, she cried in a hoarse voice into the gathering nightfall, "Someday, there will be a day of reckoning for this. *C'est la guerre.* And I'll never, never surrender."

"You tell 'em, dearie," yelled the Irish woman. As Danielle and the other lifeboat occupants stared at the U-boat, a mighty force began to gather below them. Silent as a thief, a swift undersea current drew water from beneath the bobbing craft.

Danielle sensed an eerie calm.

She turned and gasped.

A wall of water, born of the wake of the *Newell-Grey Explorer,* rose high behind them.

The wave crashed down, flipping the lifeboat like a leaf. Grappling for a handhold, Danielle screamed, and then plunged into the swirling current. The lifeboat completed its airborne arch, and an oar hurtled toward her. She tried to twist away, but it cracked her on her head, stunning her to the core.

Her moans for help were muffled as she sank into the frigid depths. She flailed about, desperate to swim the short distance to the surface, but her efforts only sucked her farther into the unrelenting sea. At last, she felt nothing but the icy claws of the Atlantic. Her breath gave way and she slipped into darkness.

Vintage Perfumes

To continue reading *Scent of Triumph*, visit your favorite retailer or order online. Also available in ebook and audiobook editions.

For Book Clubs
Scent of Triumph is a popular book club selection. Turn the page to discover book club questions that are included in the back of each copy of *Scent of Triumph* and as online downloads for audiobook listeners.

Additionally, look for *Flawless*, the first in Jan Moran's contemporary novel series set in the perfume, beauty, and fashion industries, *The Love California* series.

Scent of Triumph Book Club Discussion

The questions below are designed to facilitate discussions in book clubs. These are also available online to download at www.JanMoran.com.

1. In the beginning of the story, Danielle is constrained by societal values, but as the story progresses, she shuns convention. Why do you think her beliefs and behavior changed?

2. Women's career roles in history underwent seismic shifts during World War II. Do you think that Danielle's motivation for business was external, internal, or both? Why?

3. How would today's modern communications of mobile phones, email, and satellite media have changed this story? The relationship between Danielle and Jon? The war itself?

4. Danielle experienced life through her sense of smell. What are your favorite olfactory observations in this story?

5. How does Danielle's keen sense of smell add to setting and characterization?

6. Danielle and Max make the distinction between Germany and the Nazi party. How does this conflict affect their relationship? How do politics affect other relationships in the families?

7. When Danielle is launching her perfume line at Bullock's Wilshire in Los Angles, she realizes she feels like an American. What do you think she meant by that? Do you have any stories of immigration in your own family?

8. Do you know what year women in your country gained the right to vote? The right to own property? Can you imagine how having new access to these rights might have motivated women? Why or why not?

9. Danielle never gives up hope of finding her son, and senses that he still lives. Do you think parents have a sixth sense about the well-being of their children?

10. As an entrepreneur, what were Danielle's challenges and keys to success? Do you have any entrepreneurial ambitions, or have you ever started a new venture? Do you know where might you find advice in your community or network?

Scent of Triumph AromaTrack

In writing *Scent of Triumph*, I created an aromatrack to accompany the story and heighten the experience, just as movie soundtracks enhance stories with a related sensory experience. I often set the scene and my writing space with true-to-the-period perfume and music. Try it yourself when you read *Scent of Triumph* or any historical fiction.

The European Conflict Begins
Women
    Normandie by Jean Patou (1935)
    Mitsouko (1919)
    Shalimar by Guerlain (1925)
    Chanel No. 5 (1921)
    Cocktail by Jean Patou (1930)
    Habanita by Molinard (1921)
    Après L'Ondée by Guerlain (1906)
    Narcisse Noir by Caron (1912)
    Quelques Fleurs L'Original by Houbigant (1912)

Men
    Spanish Leather by Geo. F. Trumper (1902)
    Chanel Eau de Cologne (1929) Unisex

Mouchoir de Monsieur by Guerlain (1904)
Jicky by Guerlain (1889)
Eau de Cologne du Coq (1894) Unisex
Dunhill for Men (1934)

Arriving in America
Women
Tabac Blond by Caron (1919)
Vol de Nuit by Guerlain (1933)
En Avion by Caron (1932)
Bandit by Robert Piguet (1944)
Blue Grass by Elizabeth Arden (1934)

Men
Old Spice by Shulton (1937)
Lavanda Imperiale by Santa Maria Novella (1937)
Madrigal by Molinard (1935)

Return to Europe
Women
Nuit de Noël by Caron (1922)
Cuir de Russie by Chanel (1927)
Pour Une Femme de Caron (1942)

Men
Spanish Leather by Geo. F. Trumper (1902)
Portugal by Geo. F. Trumper (1938)

Contact Us

Thank you for reading *Vintage Perfumes*. For updates about new releases, visit www.JanMoran.com and join Jan's VIP mailing list.

Let us know how you liked *Vintage Perfumes*; we'd love to hear from you. For book club meetings, Skype events, personal appearances, or media interviews, contact Jan directly on her website.

Follow Jan on Twitter @janmoran, Facebook, Goodreads, Bookbub, and on other social media.

Did you enjoy this book? A nice review is a cherished "thank you" to the author. If you liked this book, please leave a short review where you purchased this book, or on Goodreads, for your fellow readers. Thank you!

About the Author

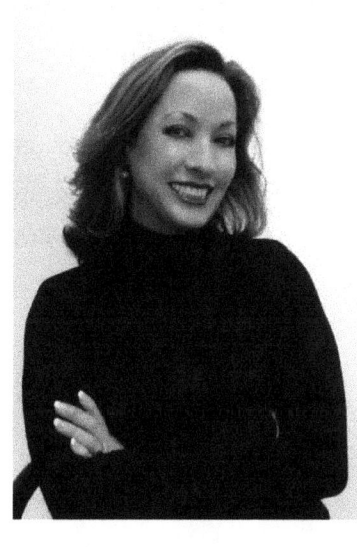

JAN MORAN is a writer and entrepreneur living in southern California.

Jan has been featured in and written for many prestigious media outlets, including CNN, Wall Street Journal, Women's Wear Daily, Allure, InStyle, O Magazine, Cosmopolitan, Elle, and Costco Connection, and has spoken before numerous groups, such as San Diego State University, Fashion Group International, The Fragrance Foundation, and The American Society of Perfumers.

She is the founder and creator of Scentsa, a touch-screen software program for retailers and brands. The fragrance and skincare programs debuted at Sephora stores as the Fragrance IQ and SkinIQ in the US, Canada, France, Mexico, Brazil, and Denmark. Scentsa was sold to Sephora.

She is a graduate of the Harvard Business School, the University of Texas at Austin, and the University of California at Los Angeles Writers Program.

Aside from Jan's professional life, a few of her favorite things include a good cup of coffee, dark chocolate, history, traveling anywhere, spas, and a warm sunny beach. Jan is originally from Austin, Texas, and a trace of a drawl still survives to this day, although she has lived in Southern California for years. She is passionate about writing and entrepreneurship.

She loves to hear from readers, and can be found on Twitter @janmoran, or walking on the beach, dreaming up another book. Say hello and sign up for her Readers Club to learn of new releases.

Write to Jan at:

Jan Moran
Sunny Palms Press
9663 Santa Monica Blvd, STE 1158, Beverly Hills, CA, USA

www.sunnypalmspress.com
www.JanMoran.com

www.ingramcontent.com/pod-product-compliance
Lightning Source LLC
Chambersburg PA
CBHW051531020426
42333CB00016B/1869